ADHD Mastery
for Adults

Simple Steps to Manage Time, Reduce Overwhelm,
and Build Lifelong Skills—Even if You Struggle to Focus

Kate Winslow

ISBN: 978-1-923422-03-2

Disclaimer:
The information in this book is for educational and entertainment purposes and is not intended as legal, financial, medical, or professional advice. While efforts have been made to ensure accuracy as of 2024, no guarantees are made regarding the content's completeness or applicability.

Readers should consult licensed professionals before applying any techniques or strategies discussed. The author and publisher are not responsible for any outcomes, losses, or consequences resulting from the use of this book's information.

Table of Contents

Introduction

You begin a task with focus, but before you can make progress, your attention is hijacked. A phone buzzes with a notification, tomorrow's deadline creeps into your thoughts, and suddenly, the chatter of colleagues, the bubbling of the water dispenser, and the constant ringing of telephones around you.

...Before you know it, you've lost track of time, where you were, and what you were doing.

For most people, this might happen occasionally on a busy day. But for individuals with ADHD, this can be a frequent and overwhelming experience, making even simple tasks feel like an uphill battle.

ADHD is often reduced to a stereotype of distraction or hyperactivity, but the reality is far more complex. Imagine your mind as a crowded room, where every detail—a ticking clock, flickering light, or stray thought—competes for attention. For individuals with ADHD, this mental clutter isn't situational; it's constant, weaving itself into every aspect of life, from managing responsibilities to maintaining relationships.

The good news? There are ways to manage and navigate these moments.

This handbook is designed to demystify ADHD, offering practical insights and strategies for anyone living with or supporting someone with the condition. ADHD exists on a spectrum, with each individual experiencing unique challenges, whether it's inattention, hyperactivity, or impulsivity. While living with ADHD can feel like swimming against the tide, effective tools and strategies can make the journey smoother—and more empowering.

Through years of research and personal experience, I've compiled this guide to share the most practical techniques for thriving with ADHD. Inside, you'll find tools to improve time management, organization, relationships, self-esteem, and overall well-being.

The book is divided into easy-to-follow chapters, each addressing a key aspect of living with ADHD:

- **Understanding ADHD**: Myths, symptoms, and deeper insights.
- **Time Management**: Tools to reduce procrastination and stay on track.
- **Organization**: Tips for simplifying your home, work, and life.
- **Relationships**: Strategies to improve communication and connection.
- **Self-Esteem**: Building confidence by embracing your unique strengths.
- **Work and Career**: Excelling in your career while managing challenges.
- **Health and Well-being**: Prioritizing your mental and physical health.

Whether you've just been diagnosed or have lived with ADHD for years, you may have felt misunderstood, overwhelmed, or exhausted. This book is here to change that, providing clarity, guidance, and hope.

You have the ability to thrive with ADHD. Let this handbook be your guide as we navigate the challenges, celebrate your strengths, and work toward a fulfilling, empowered life.

–Kate Winslow

You are not here to make others understand you.
You are here to understand yourself.

– Kristen Butler

Chapter 1

Understanding ADHD
and the Spectrum

ADHD exists on a spectrum, meaning that everyone with the condition experiences it differently. For some, symptoms may be mild and manageable, while for others, they can be more intense and disruptive. This variability makes ADHD a highly individualized experience, shaped by the severity of symptoms and the unique challenges they present.

To better understand these differences, researchers and psychologists have categorized ADHD into varying levels and types, helping to provide a framework for understanding the condition.

However, beyond these classifications, learning how ADHD develops and affects the brain can offer valuable insights into managing it effectively.

In this chapter, we'll explore the complexities of the ADHD spectrum, uncover the neurological foundations of the condition, and examine how it arises.

1.1 The ADHD Spectrum

An important aspect of ADHD that you need to be aware of is the fact that ADHD is not a condition that is easily categorized or identified *immediately*. It exists on a spectrum, which means it manifests differently for everyone.

Different persons with ADHD cannot experience this condition in the exact same way, and their strengths and challenges vary widely depending on multiple factors ranging from neurological differences, environment, and personal circumstances.

Primary Types of ADHD

Currently, there are three clinically recognized primary types and presentations of ADHD and the specific symptoms experienced by individuals, according to the categorization of the DSM-5.

1. **Predominantly Inattentive Presentation**: This type is characterized by symptoms of inattention, such as difficulty sustaining focus, following detailed instructions, and organizing tasks. These individuals may appear forgetful, easily distracted, and often lose things necessary for tasks and activities.
2. **Predominantly Hyperactive-Impulsive Presentation**: This type includes symptoms of hyperactivity and impulsivity such as fidgeting, difficulty remaining seated, excessive talking, and interrupting others. Individuals of this type may act without thinking and may find trouble waiting for their turn.
3. **Combined Presentation**: This type is a combination of inattentive and hyperactive-impulsive symptoms. Individuals with combined presentation exhibit a mix of symptoms from both categories.

Despite the existence of these presentations of ADHD, it's important to remember that ADHD is a highly individualized type of mental disorder. Experiences from different people can vary significantly compared to other individuals with ADHD.

Low and High Functioning ADHD

In addition to the three primary types of ADHD, another way to understand how ADHD can impact functioning on different levels is by considering the descriptive categories: low and high-functioning ADHD.

Low-functioning ADHD refers to individuals who struggle significantly with day-to-day tasks due to severe ADHD symptoms. These challenges may include chronic disorganization, frequent missed deadlines, and even difficulties maintaining relationships or employment. This can often overlap with other mental health conditions, such as anxiety or depression, making it harder to manage symptoms without professional support.

High-functioning ADHD, on the other hand, describes individuals who have found ways to mask or manage their symptoms effectively, often appearing organized or successful to others. However, they have their own internal struggles, such as mental exhaustion, difficulty maintaining focus, and emotional dysregulation.

Their success often comes from strong coping mechanisms, external support systems, or hyperfocus on areas of personal interest. It's important to note that these terms are not clinical diagnoses but rather *descriptive* ways to understand how ADHD can impact functioning on different levels. A person can move between these categories depending on life circumstances, stress levels, and access to resources.

Seeking Consultation

Because ADHD exists on the spectrum, the need for professional intervention depends on how symptoms impact daily functioning. If you are unsure of what to check for, or if you are beginning to suspect that you might have ADHD, here are some key trigger points to consider:

1. **Severe Impairment in Daily Life**: If ADHD symptoms make it difficult to hold a job, maintain relationships, or manage basic responsibilities like paying bills or attending appointments, it's time to seek professional support.
2. **Co-Occurring Conditions**: If symptoms of anxiety, depression, or other mental health issues are present, they can exacerbate ADHD challenges. Addressing these co-occurring conditions often requires a healthcare professional's guidance.
3. **Unmanageable Emotional Dysregulation**: Frequent emotional outbursts, intense frustration, or difficulty managing stress may indicate a need for therapeutic support or medication.
4. **Chronic Procrastination or Avoidance**: If tasks pile up due to overwhelming inattention or fear of failure, a professional can provide strategies to overcome these patterns.
5. **Strained Relationships**: If ADHD symptoms create tension with family, friends, or colleagues, a therapist can help improve communication and emotional understanding.

Seeking help doesn't mean you've failed; it means you're taking proactive steps toward a better quality of life.

Professionals like psychologists, psychiatrists, and ADHD coaches can offer tailored strategies, medication, or therapy to address your specific needs.

The purpose of this spectrum is to help others acknowledge how these symptoms of varying degrees manifest and affect people's lives, as well as illustrate how ADHD is never the same for each individual.

For other developments in the research of ADHD—particularly how the ADHD spectrum overlaps with ASD (Autism Spectrum Disorder), you may check Chapter 8 of this book, which offers a brief look at the study done by researchers specializing in psychiatry and social work.

1.2 Neurological Structure and Effects

Understanding the neurobiology of ADHD is a crucial first step in supporting individuals with this condition. Below are key factors that contribute to its development.

Contrary to common belief, ADHD isn't solely about hyperactivity or inattentiveness; it is influenced by the unique wiring and functioning of the brain.

Lower Dopamine Levels

One of the key differences lies in dopamine levels, the "feel-good chemical," which heavily impacts reward and motivation. Dopamine plays a crucial role in the brain's reward system, helping to reinforce positive behaviors and sustain focus on tasks. With ADHD, dopamine levels are often lower than those without ADHD, making it harder to stay motivated and focused as everyday tasks don't provide the same rewarding sensations.

This imbalance can lead to a constant search for stimulating activities that provide the dopamine boost the brain craves.

Hypoactive Prefrontal Cortex

Beyond dopamine, we can find another significant difference in brain regions like the prefrontal cortex. This area, located at the front of your brain, is responsible for executive functions — the mental skills that help you manage time, stay organized, and make decisions. This means that the prefrontal cortex tends to be less active for those with ADHD.

Reduced activity in the prefrontal cortex can result in impaired executive functions, making it difficult to plan, prioritize, and complete tasks.

Neurochemical Disruption

Neurotransmitter activity also plays an important role in determining how our brain coordinates with our body, as these are chemicals that transmit signals between nerve cells.

The balance and transmission of these chemicals can be disrupted, which affects how efficiently different parts of the brain communicate, leading to challenges with impulse control and sustaining attention. This would be like watching a movie where the audio and video are out of sync. That's how the ADHD-affected brain can feel when trying to process information.

1.3 Developmental Factors of ADHD

Before we dive deeper into this condition, it should be noted that the development of ADHD has no single cause. Current studies and research have determined that ADHD is natural in the sense that it is a recognized neurodevelopmental condition with strong genetic and biological underpinnings.

While environmental factors, including upbringing, can influence the severity and manifestation of symptoms, they do not solely cause ADHD. This means that a complex interaction or combination of multiple factors can only increase the *likelihood* of developing the condition.

Genetic Factors

Studies have shown that ADHD often runs in the family—it's been estimated to be highly heritable, with suggestions that about 80% of the risk is genetic. And it's not caused by one single gene, either—research identified several genes associated with ADHD—making it a complex interplay of multiple genetic factors.

Let's say if a parent has ADHD, there's a 50% chance that their child will also have it. If an older sibling has ADHD, the risk is around 30%, and so on, and can also suggest that ADHD is also a biological condition.

Environmental Influences

Environmental influences, which include negative psychological and physical factors, should be considered. This would mean the following factors have the potential to increase the risk of developing ADHD:

- **Prenatal exposure** to toxins during pregnancy, such as lead, alcohol, and smoking.
- **Immediate environment** includes Socioeconomic status, neighborhood safety, and access to resources.
- **Early childhood experiences**, including exposure to stress or trauma, can also exacerbate symptoms. This psychological factor is usually caused by the other factors mentioned in this list.

Environmental factors and genetic predispositions influence how ADHD manifests in each individual. Being aware of these factors may explain why your symptoms fluctuate or intensify under certain, more specific, conditions, especially due to psychological stress and traumatic experiences.

Psychosocial Factors

Psychosocial factors can heavily influence expression and management. These are factors that revolve around family, education, and social experiences:

- **Family Environment**: Children raised in structured, nurturing, and supportive family environments tend to fare better in managing their ADHD symptoms. Factors such as parental involvement, positive parenting practices, and consistent regulation of routines can help mitigate the impact of ADHD.
- **Educational Settings**: Schools and teachers play a significant role in shaping the experiences of children with ADHD. Adapted teaching methods, individualized education plans (IEPs), and supportive learning environments can enhance academic performance and reduce stress.
- **Social Interactions**: Peer relationships and social skills training are vital. The more negative social experiences or bullying a person with ADHD goes through, the more it can exacerbate symptoms and contribute to emotional difficulties.

In understanding these internal factors that affect the brain, the functional differences between ADHD-affected and non-ADHD brains become clear—extending to everyday activities that involve executive functions, impulse control issues, and sustaining attention.

Recognizing that these challenges stem from the brain's structure and function, you can begin to approach those with ADHD with more compassion and strategic interventions.

1.4 Emotional Dysregulation and ADHD

Emotional dysregulation is another common challenge that may be associated with ADHD, referring to the difficulty in managing and responding to emotional experiences.

Those affected may find themselves suddenly engulfed in anger or irritation over minor inconveniences, or they might even experience rapid mood swings that leave them feeling emotionally exhausted.

Such intense emotions can arise without warning, making it challenging to maintain a sense of equilibrium—situations, such as those that can frustrate you unexpectedly (e.g., losing your keys), can escalate into a full-blown outburst, leaving you and those around you bewildered and hurt. These types of episodes can make daily interactions vulnerable to tension and misunderstanding.

These emotional regulation issues inevitably spill over into personal and professional relationships as well. In personal relationships, misunderstandings and conflicts can become a regular occurrence; your partner might not understand why you react so strongly to seemingly insignificant issues, leading to arguments and strain.

The unpredictability of your emotional responses can make others feel like they're walking on eggshells, unsure of how to support you.

And at work, these emotional fluctuations can be equally disruptive. A colleague's offhand comment might trigger an intense reaction, causing friction and potentially damaging professional relationships. The inability to regulate emotions can make teamwork challenging, as others may perceive you as volatile or unreliable—leading to unwanted consequences in professional settings.

As emotional regulation can be demanding for those with ADHD, severe burnout is an all-too-common experience. Once you're burnt out, your ability to maintain focus and attention to tasks will be heavily affected, which can hinder you from finishing any of your projects and assignments.

Scientific insights shed light on the neurological basis of emotional dysregulation in ADHD. Research has shown that the amygdala, the brain's emotional center, functions differently in individuals with ADHD. The amygdala is responsible for processing emotions such as fear, anxiety, and anger.

In people with ADHD, this region can be hyperactive, leading to exaggerated emotional responses. Additionally, studies on emotional processing reveal that the frontal cortex, which helps regulate and interpret emotions, often shows decreased activity in ADHD. This imbalance between the amygdala and the frontal cortex contributes to difficulties in managing emotions.

Understanding these neurological pillars can provide validation and a sense of relief, knowing that these challenges are rooted in brain function rather than personal failure.

1.5 ADHD from Childhood to Adulthood

As children with ADHD grow into adulthood, symptoms often evolve—the hyperactivity that may have characterized their childhood years tends to diminish over time, and instead, inattentiveness becomes more pronounced.

This shift can be misleading; while the child who couldn't sit still in class might now appear calm, the internal struggle to maintain focus persists. Alongside this, new challenges emerge. Issues like organizing tasks and managing time become more apparent, which creates a perfect storm of frustration and inefficiency, making everyday activities feel like an uphill battle.

Transitioning from teenagers to young adults, where professional development becomes their main focus, can pose a significant challenge as well. Because higher education demands a level of self-discipline and organization, the progression from high school to college often results in a loss of structured support, making it harder to manage assignments and study schedules.

Later on, as young adults in work settings, the structured school environment is replaced by the often chaotic and demanding world of work. In adulthood, work-related stress and time management challenges often intensify, with looming deadlines and the constant demand for multitasking making task prioritization feel overwhelming. A high-pressure work environment can lead to missed deadlines, strained colleague relationships, and even job instability in extreme cases.

The pressure to perform can be immense, creating a cycle of stress and underachievement. As this is the case for most workplaces, having workplace accommodations such as flexible schedules, quiet workspaces, and the ability to take breaks can make a significant difference. Although some employers may lack a full understanding or delay in providing accommodations, workplace awareness around mental health and productivity strategies is growing.

Many individuals are effectively advocating for themselves and discovering creative ways to excel in their careers, even in settings that may not immediately offer the support they need.

1.6 Recent Research and Emerging Insights

There have been several studies that have been conducted to take deeper investigations into how a brain with ADHD works.

These ranged from neurological, genetic, and longitudinal studies, as well as comparative studies with developmental disorders.

Neurological Studies

One of the most significant strides has been in neuroimaging. Modern imaging techniques like MRI and PET scans have allowed scientists to observe the ADHD brain in unprecedented detail, with studies revealing distinctive patterns in brain structure and connectivity, such as how research has shown that individuals with ADHD often exhibit differences in white matter fiber bundles and gray matter density.

Findings such as these help us understand why certain brain regions, such as the frontal lobes and temporal gyri, function differently in those with ADHD. Such insights not only validate the experiences of those living with ADHD but also pave the way for more targeted and effective interventions.

Genetic Research

Genetic research has also provided valuable insights. ADHD is highly heritable, with studies indicating that about 80% of the risk is genetic. Genome-wide association studies (GWAS) have identified several genetic loci associated with ADHD, though these explain only a small fraction of the genetic variance.

This brings us to an intriguing concept known as "hidden heritability," which suggests that there are still many genetic factors yet to be discovered. Polygenic risk scores (PRS) are emerging as a potential tool for predicting ADHD-related traits and comorbidities. These scores combine data from multiple genetic markers to estimate an individual's genetic predisposition to ADHD. While not yet ready for clinical use, PRS could eventually play a role in personalized ADHD management.

Observational Findings

In terms of longitudinal studies, these have provided valuable insights into the long-term outcomes for adults with ADHD; these studies track individuals over extended periods, revealing how ADHD symptoms and their impact evolve.

One key finding is that early intervention can significantly improve outcomes. It shows that children who receive timely and appropriate treatment often experience better academic performance, social relationships, and overall quality of life. As for adults, the persistence of symptoms can vary—some find that their symptoms diminish over time, while others continue to face challenges.

Possible Treatments and Therapies

Innovative treatments and therapies are continually being developed, offering new hope for those with ADHD. Recent advancements in medication have led to the development of new medications with fewer side effects and longer-lasting effects, which provide more consistent symptom management throughout the day.

Virtual reality (VR) is another promising area, with potential applications in immersive therapy sessions that can help individuals practice social skills and emotional regulation in a controlled environment.

Personalized medicine is another frontier with great potential. This approach involves tailoring treatments to an individual's unique genetic, environmental, and lifestyle factors.

The use of pharmacogenomics—the study of how genes affect a person's response to drugs—illustrates this potential, leading to more precise medication choices, minimizing side effects, and maximizing benefits.

By considering and understanding these variables and long-term patterns, healthcare providers can develop more effective and personalized treatment plans that meet the specific needs of individuals at different life stages.

Chapter 2

Common Cognitive Challenges

Navigating daily life with ADHD often means encountering obstacles that others might not fully understand. Tasks pile up, time seems to slip away unnoticed, and even the simplest routines can feel overwhelming. These struggles stem from specific cognitive challenges that are part of living with ADHD.

In this chapter, we'll delve into key areas where these challenges arise: executive function deficits, time blindness, working memory issues, focus and attention difficulties, and organizational problems. By understanding these core hurdles, we can shed light on their impact and begin to explore actionable strategies for managing them effectively.

2.1 Executive Function Deficits

Imagine trying to navigate a complex maze without a map or compass—this is what life can feel like for anyone facing challenges with focus, organization, or executive function.

Managing everyday activities and achieving long-term goals are part of our executive functions, which are the mental skills that encompass several cognitive processes such as planning and prioritizing, working memory, and cognitive flexibility:

- **Planning and prioritizing** help you decide what needs to be done first and how to tackle it; for example, when preparing a meal, you must plan the steps and prioritize tasks like chopping vegetables before cooking.
- **Working memory** involves holding and manipulating information over short periods, such as remembering a phone number long enough to dial it.
- **Cognitive flexibility** allows you to adapt to new situations and think about multiple concepts simultaneously, which is essential when switching between tasks or coming up with creative solutions.

Once the brain is affected by certain factors, which are not ADHD-exclusive (e.g. significant stress, neurological conditions, or aging), executive functions are then impaired, and its impact on daily life can be profound. There could be an increased and constant difficulty in organizing tasks, to the point where you might even find yourself staring at a cluttered desk, unsure where to begin. This disorganization can also extend to other activities that require you to focus, such as household chores and handling work projects.

Trouble with time management can be another common issue, wherein you might underestimate how long tasks will take, leading to missed deadlines and last-minute rushes. This struggle with time can create a perpetual state of stress and anxiety, making it even harder to focus and be productive.

Identifying executive function deficits is the first step toward improvement, with valuable tools like self-assessment questionnaires that are readily available online; these often include questions about daily habits and behaviors, helping you pinpoint specific areas of difficulty.

Behavioral indicators also provide clues—these can manifest from consistently losing items, forgetting appointments, or struggling to follow multi-step instructions, which can signal executive function challenges. The earlier you recognize these signs, the better you can understand your strengths and weaknesses.

2.2 Time Blindness

Time blindness is when your internal clock is out of sync with the rest of the world, making it difficult to gauge the passage of time accurately—this phenomenon can lead to chronic lateness, missed deadlines, and a perpetual state of playing catch-up.

Time blindness isn't just about losing track of hours; people with ADHD tend to get caught up in the present moment, making it hard to plan or act for future benefits and consequences.

The next few sections will explain how time blindness affects their lifestyle.

Routine Disruptions

Starting your morning routine can be particularly challenging for individuals with ADHD. You might intend to spend only a few minutes on a task, but before you know it, an hour has gone by. This would often leave you rushing to get ready and out the door, forcing you to start the day in a state of stress and disarray. The inconsistency and lack of structure in the morning can set a chaotic tone for the rest of the day.

Planning evening activities can also be difficult—without a clear sense of time, it's easy to spend too long on one activity, inadvertently cutting into time meant for other tasks or relaxation. This can lead to late nights and inadequate rest, impacting your ability to function effectively the next day. The cycle of poor time management continues to affect both your productivity and well-being.

Difficulties in a Professional Setting

At work, time blindness can lead to missed deadlines or last-minute rushes to complete tasks. This can create significant stress and negatively impact your performance and reputation. The constant pressure of trying to catch up can make it difficult to deliver quality work, and colleagues or supervisors might start to view you as unreliable, even if you are putting in considerable effort.

Meanwhile, managing work hours effectively becomes particularly tough for individuals with ADHD. Overestimating how much can be done in a day often leads to incomplete tasks and mounting work pressure. This misjudgment can cause a perpetual backlog of work, making it hard to keep up with new tasks and increasing the overall stress and anxiety associated with your job.

Social and Personal Life

Being constantly late for appointments or social engagements can strain relationships with friends, family, and colleagues. This lateness can be perceived as a lack of respect for others' time, even though it's not intentional.

Over time, these repeated incidents can lead to frustration and disappointment, affecting your social bonds and potentially causing conflicts. Hobbies and personal projects often suffer as time slips away unnoticed. You may start with enthusiasm, only to find that days or weeks have gone by without making significant progress. This can lead to a growing list of unfinished projects and a feeling of being unaccomplished, which can be discouraging and impact your overall sense of well-being.

Academic Struggles

Students with ADHD often struggle to stick to study schedules, resulting in uneven distribution of study time. They might spend excessive time on subjects of interest while neglecting others, or conversely, rush through material without proper understanding. This inconsistency can lead to gaps in knowledge and preparedness, affecting overall academic performance.

Time blindness can also cause assignments to be started late or rushed, significantly impacting the quality of work. The last-minute efforts to complete tasks can lead to increased stress and subpar academic outcomes. This pattern of procrastination and cramming can become a recurring issue, further complicating the academic experience for students with ADHD.

Overall Well-being

Constantly feeling like you're running out of time or playing catch-up can lead to chronic stress and anxiety. This ongoing pressure can take a toll on mental health, exacerbating ADHD symptoms and creating a cycle of stress that is hard to break. Feeling like you would never be able to fully catch up can be overwhelming, and this can be very detrimental to your overall well-being.

As for sleep, the inconsistent perception of time can disrupt sleep schedules, leading to insufficient or irregular sleep. Poor sleep quality and irregular sleep patterns can further exacerbate ADHD symptoms, making it even more challenging to manage daily tasks and responsibilities. This lack of proper rest can affect mood, cognitive function, and overall health. Recognizing these patterns is the first step in finding ways to manage time more effectively and reduce the associated stress.

2.3 Working Memory Challenges

Working memory issues can be another significant cognitive challenge for individuals with ADHD, affecting their ability to retain and manipulate information over short periods.

This can make everyday tasks more difficult to manage and often leads to feelings of frustration and perceptions of unreliability, such as:

- **Forgetting Important Details:** Individuals often forget crucial parts of conversations or instructions, leading to misunderstandings and incomplete tasks.
- **Losing Track of Belongings:** Frequently misplacing everyday items like keys or important documents can cause delays and additional stress.
- **Struggling with Task Completion:** Multi-step tasks and projects can feel overwhelming, resulting in difficulty completing them efficiently.
- **Inability to Retain Information:** In the academic and professional setting, remembering lectures or meetings can be challenging, affecting performance and reliability.
- **Forgetting social commitments:** Details from personal conversations can strain relationships and cause feelings of disconnection.

Understanding these working memory challenges highlights their pervasive impact on daily life, from managing tasks and responsibilities to maintaining relationships.

2.4 Focus and Attention Issues

Maintaining focus and attention can be particularly challenging for individuals with ADHD. Distractibility is a constant companion, with both external stimuli and internal thoughts pulling attention away from tasks, making it hard to complete tasks efficiently and can lead to mistakes and oversight.

Diffused Thinking

When one mentions *ADHD*, one may think that it means having a "complete lack of attention and focus"—which is a misguided belief. On the contrary, those with ADHD often pay attention to *everything*—all at once.

It is incorrect to assume that those with ADHD are "attention deficit," as this suggests the idea that they have a *complete* lack of attention. Instead, their attention to every single detail simultaneously is called having diffused thinking, which is often described by those with ADHD as scattered or jumping from one thing to another quickly, which leads to increased difficulty in focusing on a single task.

Diffused thinking is commonly separated into two traits: "constant distractibility," a hallmark of ADHD, where noises, visual distractions, and other environmental factors can easily divert attention. For example, the sound of a coworker's conversation or notifications on a phone can interrupt focus on a task. Internal thoughts, such as racing thoughts and daydreaming, also pull attention away from immediate tasks, making it difficult to stay on track.

And then there's "difficulty sustaining attention," especially on repetitive or uninteresting tasks, which can quickly make mundane activities unbearable, leading to frequent task-switching and incomplete work. For instance, routine paperwork or data entry can feel intolerable, resulting in procrastination and chaos. The inability to sustain attention often leads to starting multiple projects but finishing few, contributing to a cluttered and chaotic environment.

Hyperfocus and Hyperfixation

Hyperfocus allows for intense concentration on activities of interest, sometimes for hours without noticing time passing. While this can be beneficial for productivity in certain areas, it often results in the neglect of other important tasks and responsibilities.

During periods of hyperfocus, everyday obligations such as meals, appointments, or deadlines might be overlooked, leading to negative consequences in personal and professional life.

Hyperfixation, however, is *similar* to hyperfocus, but it lasts much longer—an obsessive interest in particular areas. The impact on daily life is significant. In a work setting, distractibility and difficulty sustaining attention can result in missed deadlines, lower productivity, and potential conflicts with colleagues or supervisors. For students, it can be challenging to focus during lectures or study sessions, all of which could lead to lower academic performance and increased frustration.

Additionally, distractibility can affect personal relationships, as missing out on important details during conversations can cause misunderstandings and feelings of disconnection.

2.5 Organizational Problems

Organizational skills are often impaired in individuals with ADHD, leading to both physical and mental clutter. This clutter can create a sense of overwhelm and significantly hinder productivity.

Physical and Mental Clutter

Physical clutter is a common issue. Living spaces, such as rooms and living areas, may become cluttered with items left out or disorganized. This can make it difficult to find things when needed and create a chaotic environment that adds to stress. Similarly, workspaces often become crowded with papers, supplies, and personal items; this level of disorganization can reduce efficiency and increase the time spent searching for necessary materials.

Mental clutter is equally challenging. Keeping track of multiple tasks, deadlines, and commitments can feel overwhelming, leading to information overload. This mental clutter can cause forgetting important details and feeling mentally fatigued.

Additionally, having too many options or tasks to manage can result in decision paralysis. This can lead to inaction and a buildup of tasks.

Long-Term Planning and Multitasking

Difficulty planning ahead compounds these issues. Long-term projects, without clear steps and organization, can feel unattainable. The lack of a structured plan can make it challenging to make consistent progress, leading to procrastination and missed deadlines.

Similarly, setting and achieving long-term goals can be difficult without effective organizational strategies, making goals feel out of reach and creating a lack of direction.

Another difficulty faced by those with ADHD is the increased challenge of multi-tasking or task switching, which also presents a significant challenge. Moving from one task to another can be difficult, leading to wasted time and a feeling of being stuck. This inefficiency can disrupt the flow of work and reduce overall productivity.

Additionally, adapting to changes and managing multiple responsibilities can be challenging, leading to a sense of being overwhelmed and unable to keep up with demands.

Chapter 3

Enhancing Executive Functions

Executive functions are the mental skills that enable us to plan, organize, and complete tasks. For individuals with ADHD, these processes can often feel like uphill battles, impacting memory, focus, decision-making, and task management. While these challenges can disrupt daily life, they are not insurmountable.

In this chapter, we'll explore practical ways to strengthen executive functions and regain control over your daily routines. From memory aids and focus techniques to planning, goal setting, and progress tracking, you'll discover actionable strategies to overcome common hurdles. We'll also dive into managing impulsivity, prioritizing tasks effectively, and leveraging modern tools like apps to stay organized—addressing these areas will equip you with the skills and resources needed to navigate life with greater clarity and confidence.

3.1 Memory and Focus Aids and Techniques

Memory and focus challenges are common experiences for many people. However, for those with ADHD, depending on the severity of symptoms, it can be twice as frustrating when short-term memory slips. The combination of the inability to focus on information and retain them in memory can become problematic. These moments can disrupt daily life and make tasks feel more challenging.

Working memory, which allows us to manage and manipulate information over short periods, can be compromised, which can make following multi-step instructions a daunting task.

Finding difficulty with recalling and focusing on small or important tasks under stress is another common issue; the more anxious or overwhelmed you become, your brain's ability to retrieve information plummets, which could lead to embarrassing moments, like forgetting a colleague's name during a meeting or missing a crucial deadline. Thankfully, there are many ways to manage memory and focus challenges.

Building Routines

Routines can be your memory and focus anchor, especially if you have ADHD. These provide structure and predictability in an otherwise unpredictable world, which can significantly impact your mental health and productivity. Knowing what to expect next will decrease stress levels and make daily chores and errands more manageable and easier to remember and focus on.

An established routine will allow you to build better habits, making it easier to perform daily activities without overthinking them. By creating a consistent daily routine, you can improve your overall well-being, leading to better sleep, healthier eating habits, and increased focus. Creating a personalized routine starts with identifying your key daily activities. List everything you need to do in a day.

Your routine can look as simple as this:

- Waking up early in the morning and shower
- Go for a walk (4km)
- Prepare and eat meals
- Brush your teeth after an hour
- Do work tasks/household chores
- (Any leisurely activity such as playing video games, watching your favorite shows, etc.)
- Prepare for bed and sleep for the day.

You can prioritize these activities based on their importance and urgency.

Then, once you have these listed down, you can begin establishing a more consistent wake-up and bedtime schedule, especially since regular sleep patterns are necessary for managing ADHD symptoms. Having a consistent routine can help regulate your internal clock, making it easier to fall asleep and wake up at the same time each day.

Following your routine religiously will eventually help you reduce the likelihood of getting sidetracked. Even though keeping a consistent routine can be challenging, there are some strategies that can help:

- **Habit-tracking apps:** These apps (found on your preferred app stores) can be incredibly useful. These allow you to set daily goals and track your progress, providing visual reminders and rewards for staying on track—some even gamify the habit-tracking experience for those who prefer a more engaging yet productive way of maintaining your healthier routine habits throughout the day.

- **Set Daily Reminders:** You can set alarms on your phone or use a physical planner to prompt you to start and stop activities at the right times.
- **Accountability partners:** These can be a close friend or family member who can check in with you regularly, offering encouragement and support. This external accountability can motivate you to stick to your routine, even on challenging days.

However, life can still be unpredictable despite taking measures to organize your day, so your routine must be flexible enough to accommodate changes. Because of how unpredictable life can be, it's necessary to realize when a routine isn't working, and adjusting it is crucial.

Sometimes, routine fatigue can slowly set in when the same activities become monotonous or overwhelming. You can prevent this by periodically reviewing your routine and making the necessary adjustments. If you find that certain tasks consistently cause stress or they somehow take longer than expected, pause and consider re-evaluating how they fit into your schedule. Routine planning flexibility means being open to change and willing to experiment with different approaches.

Suppose you usually exercise in the morning but find it hard to get motivated, try shifting your workout to the afternoon. In that case, small adjustments like that can make a significant difference in maintaining a routine that works for you.

Routines are not static; they evolve with your needs and circumstances. Be patient, and give yourself grace as you develop and refine your routine. Building and maintaining a routine takes time and effort, but the benefits are well worth it.

Virtual and Physical External Aids

In this day and age, having digital calendars with reminders is indispensable. Digital calendars can sync across all your devices, ensuring you never miss an important date—this includes reminders for everything from meetings to medication times.

Another external aid you can use is a physical notebook; writing things down in a planner or small notebook (e.g., dotted, grid, ruled, blank) can help imprint information into your memory. You can jot down tasks and ideas as they come—or if you simply want to remember certain information better, you can do this by doodling, which has been proven true by Jackie Andrade, who conducted research back in 2009 on how making small sketches during class helped students recall their lessons better.

Meanwhile, sticky notes placed in strategic locations, like your bathroom mirror or computer screen, can serve as visual cues for important tasks.

Mnemonics and Acronyms

There are also memory techniques that can further bolster your recall abilities. **Mnemonics and acronyms** are useful for remembering lists or sequences.

For example, the acronym "<u>HOMES</u>" can help you recall the Great Lakes:

1. Huron
2. Ontario
3. Michigan
4. Erie
5. Superior

Visualization Techniques and Memory Palace

Visualization techniques can also be powerful—try to create vivid mental images of the information you need to remember. If you need to remember to buy milk, visualize a giant milk carton sitting on your kitchen counter.

Similar to the visualization technique, the *loci* method, or memory palace, is another effective technique, and this involves associating information with specific locations in a familiar place, like your home.

Imagine walking through your house and placing items you need to remember in different rooms. When you need to recall the information, you mentally walk through your house and "see" the items in their designated spots.

Positive Reinforcement

Another way to overcome focus and memory difficulties is to find ways to actively motivate yourself, in which positively reinforcing certain actions by setting up reward systems can be highly effective.

Set up a system where completing each task or mini-deadline earns you a small reward. Small rewards include:

- Eating your favorite snack
- Taking a short break
- Putting time into your favorite hobby

Aside from physically rewarding yourself, visualizing your end goals can also boost motivation. Picture the satisfaction you'll feel when the project is complete, or imagine the positive feedback you'll receive from your boss. This mental imagery can make the effort feel more worthwhile.

Other Digital Apps and Tools

Technology can, understandably, be a double-edged sword, being both a distraction and a solution. Thankfully, some apps can benefit your memory and focus, like "brain music" audio player apps that use auditory neuroscience for scientifically optimized music that helps you get into an improved concentration state faster.

Website blockers can help you avoid digital distractions by blocking access to time-wasting websites during work hours. Or, you can set up your device's notification control settings to limit interruptions by disabling non-essential notifications or using "*Do Not Disturb*" mode when you need to focus and build a healthier boundary between you and distracting websites (e.g., social media and video streaming sites).

Finally, we have visual timers for more focused work or hobby sessions. They are invaluable tools for combating time blindness, as making the passage of time visible can help you stay aware of how long you've been working on something, as well as making sure you don't focus *too* much on one task at a time—which could lead to disregard of other important house errands or work projects.

Set a visual timer on your desk or use a timer app on your phone; watching the time countdown can provide a sense of urgency and keep you focused.

Setting alarms for key parts of your day, such as starting and ending work, taking breaks, or transitioning between tasks, is also effective. Reminders like these can act as external prompts, helping you stay on track.

A good visual timer you can use is a Pomodoro timer, which is specifically designed to help you stay focused. It follows the Pomodoro Technique—it is set up in a way that allows you to balance your work and break sessions in an orderly and healthy way through bursts of uninterrupted focus followed by short breaks. Here's how it's usually set up—but you can adjust it according to your preference:

1. **Four 25-minute work intervals:** This is the default time for working when following the Pomodoro Technique. You can do 30 minutes if you want to.
2. **Short 5-minute break:** After each work interval, you can proceed to take 5-minute breaks that allow you to rest and stretch.
3. **Long 15–30-minute breaks:** Once you finish a round of four work intervals, you can then take a longer break of 15-30 minutes. After that, you repeat the work-rest-long rest pattern about four more times.

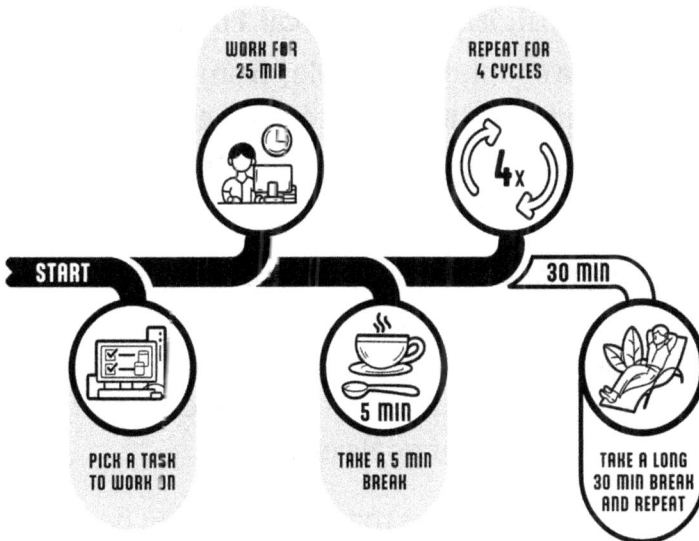

With quick work and break intervals, this approach not only combats fatigue but also provides a structured way to manage time, especially with longer or harder tasks.

3.2 Planning and Goal Setting

Planning is a key element for both short and long-term success for everyone, and this can be particularly helpful if you live with ADHD. Without a structured plan, days can sometimes feel overwhelming or disorganized.

However, having a well-thought-out plan provides direction, making tasks more manageable and your day more orderly. Knowing what to expect next will reduce any anxiety and stress before reaching your goals.

Before you get into planning, the first step is choosing the right tools once you understand your specific needs—like ease of use, portability, and preference.

Goal Setting with Digital and Physical Tools

Going back to a couple of examples from Chapter 3.1: Memory and Focus Aids and Techniques, you can essentially use digital and physical tools to start your planning and goal-setting process; both have their own pros and cons.

Digital tools, like apps, can sync across devices to ensure you have access to your plans wherever you go. You can get reminders through notifications and alarms while you're out and about. It also helps that these apps can be integrated directly into your workflow to organize your goals easily.

You will have to make sure that you keep your devices charged, however—and some apps may also have a bit of a learning curve before you can truly use them to their full potential. Not to mention the ads and premium-locked features in some apps, too.

Analog or physical tools, like planners and sticky notes, offer a more tactile engagement, which some find grounding. It's a bit more hands-on, but it does become worth the effort, especially when you write things down word-for-word, allowing you to remember your plans and goals a bit better.

The only downside is that you'll be a bit more paper-dependent, which some may find discouraging—having to keep track of journals and sticky notes—along with the mess that comes with it. It all boils down to your personal preference, however, and the key is to pick tools that *simplify* your life, not complicate it further.

Visual Categorization Methods

Once you've chosen your tools, setting up an effective organizational system is the next important step: choosing and using your visual categorization methods, which can maintain order. You can use these both digitally and physically.

Color coding is an incredibly helpful and visually intensive way to quickly categorize your plans. You can assign different colors to various tasks or categories, such as work, personal, and health. This visual differentiation can make it easier to identify and prioritize tasks.

Labeling and sorting methods are equally important; use clear, concise labels for files, bins, and folders. This reduces the time spent searching for items and helps maintain order.

Another tool for long-term planning is a vision board. A vision board is a visual representation of your goals and dreams—this can be done physically or digitally. Start by collecting *images*, *quotes*, and *other items* that inspire you.

These can come from magazines, online sources, or personal photos. Arrange them on a board in a way that resonates with you, which can be similar to a mood board that graphic designers use for pre-planning designs.

Then, place this vision board where you'll see it every day, such as in your bedroom or workspace. Seeing your goals visually can keep them at the forefront of your mind, providing daily motivation and inspiration.

Goal Management Systems

Once you've chosen your preferred medium, the next step is to choose a system you want to implement once you start planning and setting your goal.

The "one-touch" rule is a simple yet effective strategy: handle each item only once. When you pick something up, decide its fate immediately—whether it needs to be filed, trashed, or acted upon. This prevents clutter from piling up and keeps your space organized.

Another effective way to start planning once you have chosen your tool is by setting SMART goals:

- Specific
- Measurable
- Achievable
- Relevant
- Time-bound

S — **SPECIFIC**
WHO, WHAT, WHERE, AND WHY

M — **MEASURABLE**
YOU CAN'T IMPROVE WHAT YOU CAN'T MEASURE

A — **ATTAINABLE**
CHALLENGING BUT NOT IMPOSSIBLE

R — **REALISTIC**
CLOSELY CONNECTED TO YOUR GOAL

T — **TIMELY**
A DATE TO HOLD YOU ACCOUNTABLE

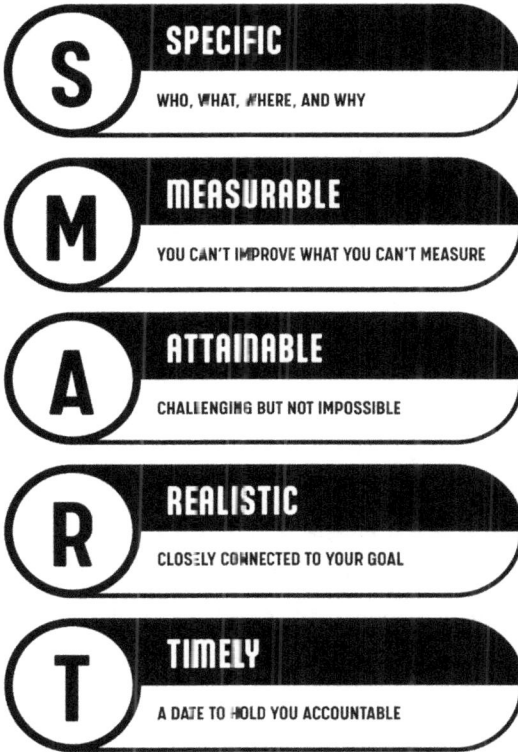

These criteria help you create clear and attainable goals. For example, instead of saying, "*I want to exercise more*," a SMART goal would be, "*I will walk for 30 minutes every morning for the next month.*" This goal is therefore:

- Specific (**walking**)
- Measurable (**30 minutes**)
- Achievable (a realistic time frame)
- Relevant (improving health)
- Time-bound (**one month**)

By setting SMART goals, you create a clear path to success, making it easier to stay focused and motivated.

Short-Term Goal Review

Once you've set your short-term goals, regularly reviewing and adjusting these goals is crucial for staying on track. Short-term goals may need to evolve over time, so scheduling a weekly or bi-weekly goal review session to assess your progress to help you evaluate what's working and what isn't can allow you to adjust your timelines and milestones as needed to stay realistic and attainable.

Long-Term Goal Review

When you do have your long-term goals, it's highly critical to set up systems for monthly goal reviews to help make your process more efficient. Use a journal or your designated digital tool to document your goals, progress, and adjustments. During your monthly review sessions, take note of any obstacles you've encountered and brainstorm solutions.

Addressing challenges before they derail your progress with this proactive approach will allow for a less problematic and more productive work session when you get right back to them.

3.3 Progress-Tracking Techniques

Once you're done with the planning and goal-setting phase, the next step is *tracking* your progress—which can be a difficult and overwhelming activity for those who have ADHD, especially when it's hard to focus on one task when you could end up focusing on *multiple at once.*

This is especially true with large-scale projects, as those can be even more overwhelming and intimidating when you look at the enormity of the tasks and feel paralyzed, not knowing where to start—making it more necessary to track your progress.

Time-Blocking Method

This is a powerful strategy for allocating specific blocks of time for different tasks throughout your day.

You can do this by dedicating an hour in the morning to checking emails, two hours for focused work, and so on.

It can look like this:

Monday
9-10 AM   Check and write emails
10 AM - 12 PM   (Focused Work Tasks)
12-1 PM   Lunch
1-2 PM   Team meeting

You can create a structured layout of the tasks that you need to do to minimize the chaos by breaking your day into manageable chunks.

Doing this improves productivity while also reducing the anxiety of not knowing what to do next.

Task Chunking

Chunking involves breaking projects into even smaller, more manageable tasks. Instead of seeing a mountain, you start to see smaller, climbable hills.

TASK CHUNKING

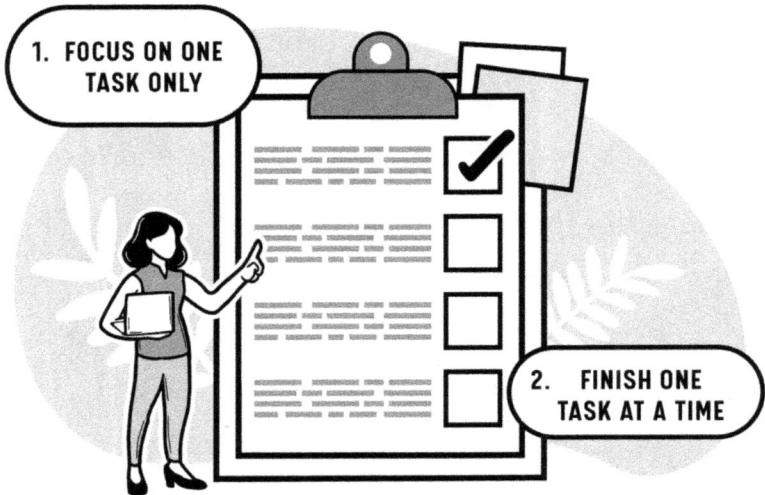

This method lets you tackle each piece individually, making the entire project less daunting. To do chunking, you need to list all the components of your project.

For this example, let's chunk tasks for *Writing–Drafting*:

1. Draft a short introduction
2. Prepare main written content with separate chapters:
   a. Chapter 1 – Topic A
   b. Chapter 2 – Topic B
   c. Chapter 3 – Topic C
3. Draft a short conclusion.

Then, take each component and break it down further. Make it as straightforward as possible:

1. Draft a short introduction
   a. Purpose of the book
   b. Goals to achieve

2. Prepare main written content with separate chapters:
    a. Chapter 1 – Topic A (applicable to other chapters)
        i. Research about Topic A
        ii. Note down research data
        iii. Create an outline for Chapter 1
            1. Introduce the topic
            2. Separate data into sub-chapters
            3. End chapter
3. Draft a short conclusion
    a. Appreciation notes
    b. Reflection and takeaways on key points

Creating step-by-step plans turns an overwhelming project into a series of smaller, achievable tasks. Each completed task provides a sense of accomplishment, which can motivate you to keep going.

Gantt Chart

Next is visualizing project timelines. A Gantt Chart can be an invaluable tool, consisting of a horizontal bar chart where each bar represents a task.

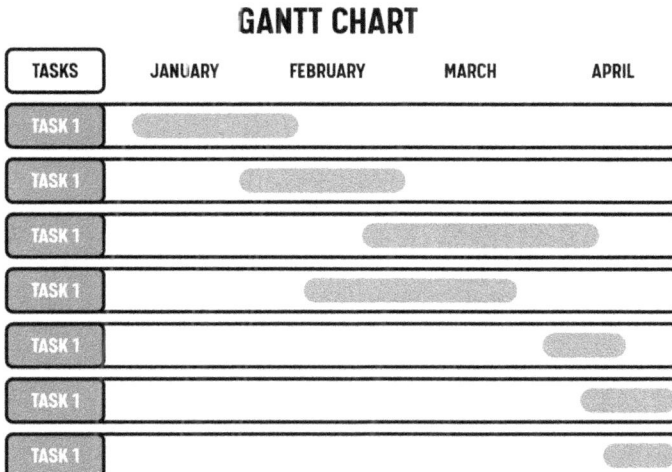

GANTT CHART

TASKS	JANUARY	FEBRUARY	MARCH	APRIL
TASK 1				
TASK 1				
TASK 1				
TASK 1				
TASK 1				
TASK 1				
TASK 1				

The length of the bar indicates the duration of the task, and the placement shows the start and end dates.

Setting up a Gantt chart helps you see the entire project at a glance. Start by listing all your tasks along the vertical axis. Then, draw horizontal bars to represent each task's duration. This visual representation makes it easier to track progress and adjust timelines as needed.

Using a Gantt chart can also help you identify dependencies between tasks. For example, you can't start the content creation phase until the research phase is complete. By visualizing these dependencies, you can plan more effectively and avoid bottlenecks. Regularly update your Gantt chart to reflect progress and any changes in timelines. This keeps you on track and ensures you're moving forward systematically.

Lastly, for prioritizing subtasks in large projects, it's always important to note that not all tasks are equally important; some are more critical than others, and properly identifying critical tasks can help you focus your energy where it's needed most.

Pareto Principle

You can start by listing all your subtasks and identifying which ones are essential for the project's success. Use the 80/20 rule, also known as the Pareto Principle, to guide you.

This principle suggests that *80% of your results come from 20% of your efforts*. Identify the 20% of tasks that will have the most significant impact on your project and prioritize them.

Once you've identified your critical tasks, rank them in order of importance. Focus on completing these tasks first before moving on to less critical ones. This approach ensures that you're making the most of your time and effort, leading to better project outcomes.

Prioritizing tasks also helps you manage your resources more effectively, ensuring that you're not spreading yourself too thin. Tracking progress on large projects is essential for staying on track and maintaining motivation. Several progress-tracking apps can help you monitor your tasks and deadlines.

These tools offer a clear overview of what's been done and what still needs attention. Regular check-ins and updates are also important. Schedule weekly or bi-weekly check-ins to review your progress and make any necessary adjustments. These check-ins provide an opportunity to address any obstacles and refine your plans.

Kanban Board

Visual progress trackers can be particularly motivating. Consider creating a progress chart or using a Kanban board to visualize your progress. A Kanban board uses columns to represent different stages of your project, such as *"To Do," "In Progress,"* and *"Completed."*

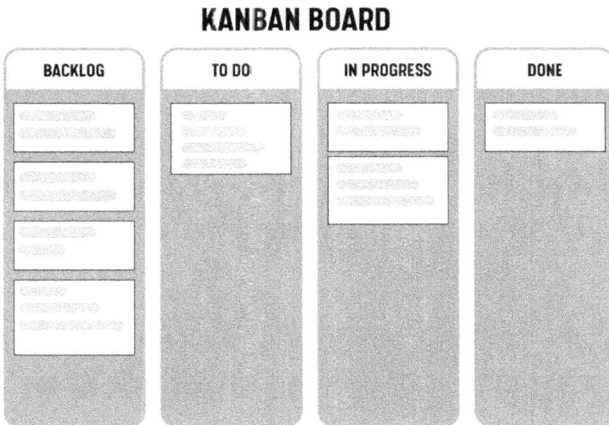

KANBAN BOARD

BACKLOG	TO DO	IN PROGRESS	DONE

As you finish up tasks one by one, you move them through each column the more you progress through your tasks. Having this visual representation would provide a clear sense of progress and can be highly motivating. It's satisfying to see tasks move from "To Do" to "Completed," and it helps you stay focused and organized.

Breaking down tasks into smaller, manageable pieces, using tools like Gantt charts, prioritizing subtasks, and tracking progress effectively can transform how you approach large projects. These strategies help you stay organized, reduce overwhelm, and maintain motivation, ensuring that you complete your projects successfully.

3.4 Task Prioritization

Effectively prioritizing tasks can significantly improve the management of ADHD symptoms, bringing more structure and ease to daily life.

By focusing on what truly matters, prioritization helps reduce the sense of overwhelm that comes with juggling multiple responsibilities, allowing you to tackle tasks with greater clarity and confidence.

Basic Prioritization

You can build to have a good overview of what you need to do for the day. Similar to what you've learned from building a routine, you can start by listing all the tasks you need to accomplish.

Unlike time-blocking, where you're effectively giving yourself a *time limit*, the purpose of this list is to prioritize tasks based on their urgency and importance—tasks with impending deadlines should take precedence over less critical ones.

Once you have your list, you can use the time-blocking method to allocate specific time slots for each task. Be realistic about how long each task will take and include buffer time for transitions and unexpected interruptions. This approach can prevent the frustration of an overpacked schedule.

There are also task management apps you can use that can allow you to create boards for different projects, add tasks, and set deadlines. These have visual layouts that can make it easy to track progress and stay organized.

Eisenhower Matrix

Next, we have the Eisenhower Matrix, which is an excellent tool for task prioritization. This matrix divides tasks into four categories:

- Urgent and important
- Important but not urgent
- Urgent but not important
- Neither urgent nor important.

By categorizing tasks this way, you can clearly see which tasks need immediate attention and which can be postponed or delegated.

Ranking tasks by importance and urgency can help you avoid the trap of spending time on less critical activities while neglecting what truly matters.

	URGENT	NOT URGENT
IMPORTANT	**DO** DO IT RIGHT AWAY	**DECIDE** SCHEDULE A TIME TO WORK ON IT LATER
NOT IMPORTANT	**DELEGATE** WHO IS THE BEST PERSON FOR THE TASK	**DELETE** REMOVE UNNECESSARY TASKS

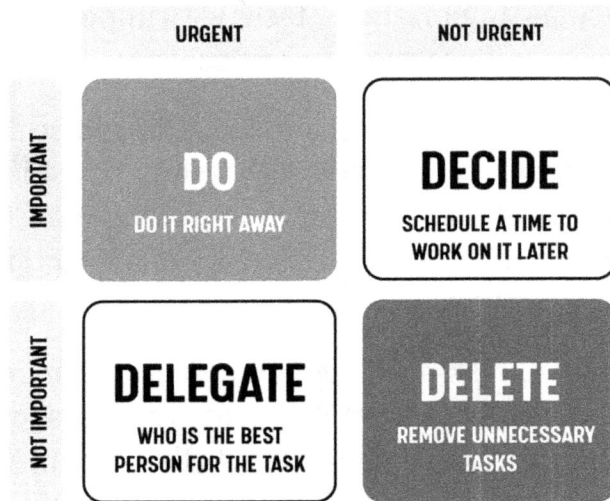

Creating an effective prioritization system involves daily and weekly task reviews. Start each day by reviewing your tasks and updating your priorities based on any new information or deadlines, and reviewing them weekly can help you take a broader look at your goals to ensure you stay on track.

Categorizing tasks can also provide clarity, where using categories like *work*, *personal*, *health*, and *leisure* to group similar tasks together can help you group, visualize, and line tasks better. This can help you see where your time is going and make more informed decisions about how to allocate it.

By consistently reviewing and categorizing your tasks, you can maintain a clear sense of direction and purpose.

Prioritization and Priority Matrix Apps

There are several tools that can assist with task prioritization. Some digital planners offer a versatile platform for organizing tasks, which allows you to create custom templates, set deadlines, and prioritize tasks using various criteria. Its flexibility makes it an excellent choice for those who need a comprehensive tool for managing multiple aspects of their life.

Priority matrix apps can also be beneficial, as these apps are specifically designed to help you implement the Eisenhower Matrix and make it easy to categorize and prioritize tasks. With tools like these, you can streamline your task management process and ensure you're focusing on what truly matters.

3.5 Decision-Making and Impulsivity

Decision-making can be challenging, especially when impulsivity takes the lead, which sometimes results in quick decisions that aren't fully thought through.

Without taking the time to weigh the pros and cons, you might find yourself making choices *at* that moment that you later wish you had reconsidered. This can create additional complexity and frustration, particularly when hindsight reveals unintended consequences.

The process of evaluating options and thinking ahead requires executive functioning, and when this process feels difficult, impulsive choices can become more frequent.

These quick decisions can impact different areas of life, from finances to relationships, potentially leaving you feeling overwhelmed and frustrated. However, with the right strategies, it's possible to regain control and make decisions with greater confidence and clarity.

DECIDE Model

Several frameworks can be highly effective in aiding in better decision-making. The DECIDE model is a structured approach that can guide you through the process.

This model consists of the following:

- Defining the problem clearly: know *exactly* what you need to decide to eliminate confusion.
- Explore the alternatives available to you: list all possible options *without* judgment.
- Consider the consequences of each alternative: think about the long and short-term impacts.
- Identify the best option based on your analysis.
- Develop a plan to implement it.
- Evaluate the decision after some time to see if it was the right choice.

This structured approach can slow down impulsive tendencies and provide a clear path to follow.

SWOT Analysis

Another useful framework is the SWOT analysis, which is most commonly used in school and work settings. This method allows you to break down a decision into manageable parts by answering the questions associated with each part:

- Strengths – *What advantages does it offer?*
- Weaknesses – *What are the potential downsides?*
- Opportunities – *What positive outcomes could result from this decision?*
- Threats – *What risks or obstacles might you face?*

By breaking down your decision into these four categories, you gain a comprehensive view of the situation, making it easier to make an informed choice.

For more complex decisions, decision matrices offer a structured way to evaluate your options. Start by setting criteria that are important to you. For example, if you're deciding on a new job, your criteria might include salary, commute time, company culture, and career growth opportunities.

Next, weigh each criterion based on its importance—if salary is the most important factor, give it a higher weight. Then, evaluate each option against these criteria, scoring them based on how well they meet each one. Finally, multiply the scores by the weights and sum them up to get a total score for each option.

The option with the highest score or heaviest weight is usually the best choice. This method provides a clear, quantitative way to compare complex options, reducing the influence of impulsivity.

Mindfulness Techniques

Finally, after learning all the strategies and structures to manage your decision-making abilities, one important set of techniques to help you make choices while reducing impulsivity is the mindfulness technique.

Deep breathing exercises can help you stay calm and centered. When faced with a decision, take a few deep breaths to clear your mind. This simple act can reduce anxiety and create a pause, giving you time to think.

The "pause and reflect" method is another effective technique—before making a decision, you should deliberately choose to take a brief pause.

During this pause, reflect on the possible outcomes and consequences. Pausing can be as short as a few seconds or as long as a few minutes, depending on the situation; the key is to create a break in the impulsive cycle, allowing for more thoughtful consideration. For more of these techniques, you can go ahead and check Chapter 6.5.

3.6 More Apps and Tools

Selecting the right apps and tools can make a world of difference for adults with ADHD—especially when most of them come with quality-of-life functions that can add to your overall productivity and routine.

The first step in this process is identifying the criteria that matter most to you. Look for apps that balance simplicity and functionality, as overly complex tools can become overwhelming, while too simplistic ones might not offer the features you need. Prioritize ease of use, intuitive interfaces, and customization options—streamline your tasks and *avoid* complicating them further.

The apps and programs listed here are some of what I have personally used for work. These are simply recommendations based on my personal preferences, but these may be of help to you, too.

Task Management Apps

Finding the right task management apps is a great starting point. *Asana* stands out for task and project management, allowing you to break down tasks into smaller, manageable steps. It also offers various views, such as lists, boards, and timelines, helping you visualize your progress. You can set deadlines, assign tasks, and track your work, making it easier to stay organized.

Todoist is another excellent option for daily tasks. Its simple interface lets you create tasks, set priorities, and track your progress. You can also integrate it with other apps, like Google Calendar, to keep everything in one place.

Note-Taking Apps

Digital note-taking tools are invaluable for organizing your thoughts and ideas. *Notion* is a versatile option, allowing you to create notes and lists and even upload or embed videos or audio. You can organize your notes into notebooks and tag them for easy retrieval.

OneNote offers a similar range of features but with a more flexible, free-form canvas. It's great for creative brainstorming, letting you mix text, images, and drawings in your notes. Both apps sync across devices, ensuring you have access to your notes wherever you go.

Automation Tools

Automation tools can significantly simplify your daily routines. *IFTTT* (*If This Then That*) allows you to create custom automation between apps and devices. For example, you can set it to automatically save email attachments to Dropbox or get a weather update every morning.

Zapier works similarly but is geared more toward business applications. It can integrate multiple apps, automating tasks like updating spreadsheets or sending reminders. These tools can save you time and reduce the mental load of repetitive tasks.

Time Trackers

Time-tracking apps are essential for improving productivity. *Toggl* is a straightforward app that lets you track work hours with a single click. You can categorize your time by projects or tasks, making it easier to see where your time goes.

RescueTime offers a more in-depth analysis, tracking the time you spend on different websites and applications. It provides detailed reports, helping you identify time sinks and adjust your habits accordingly. Both apps can help you stay accountable and make more informed decisions about how to manage your time.

Virtual Assistants

Virtual assistants like *Siri* or *Gemini* (and *Google Assistant* for some devices) can be incredibly useful for setting reminders and managing daily schedules. You can ask them to set alarms, remind you of appointments, or even create shopping lists. Assistants like these can also integrate with other apps, providing a seamless way to manage your tasks and stay organized.

For instance, you can ask Gemini or Google Assistant to add an event to your calendar or send a message, all hands-free. This can be particularly helpful when you're on the go or multitasking.

Incorporating technology into your daily routines can significantly enhance your productivity. By selecting the right tools, you can streamline your tasks, reduce overwhelm, and stay organized. Embracing these tools can help you navigate the complexities of ADHD, making it easier to stay focused and productive.

It goes without saying that using technology or apps can be a hit or miss. But as long as you find the right one that suits your needs and integrate these tools into your routine, technology can be a powerful ally in managing ADHD.

The right apps can provide structure, reduce anxiety, and help you achieve your goals more efficiently. With a well-chosen set of tools, you can enhance your executive functions and take control of your daily life.

In the next chapter, we'll explore how to navigate relationships and improve communication, providing insights and strategies to strengthen your connections with others.

Chapter 4

Managing Relationships with ADHD

Maintaining relationships is challenging for anyone, but for individuals with ADHD, these challenges can be amplified. Even in an age where awareness of mental health is growing, it can still be disheartening when your partner doesn't seem to understand what you're going through—despite your own awareness that ADHD isn't always fully understood.

Picture this: you're sitting across from your partner, explaining why you forgot an important date, only to see frustration in their eyes. You feel misunderstood, while they feel neglected—both emotions are entirely valid. Unfortunately, scenarios like these are all too common for adults with ADHD.

Symptoms such as inattentiveness or impulsivity can strain romantic relationships, making it feel like you're speaking two different languages, with neither party fully grasping the other's perspective. This disconnect can even lead to masking behaviors, where those with ADHD hide their struggles to avoid conflict.

But it doesn't have to stay this way. Understanding how ADHD affects relationships is the first step toward fostering healthier communication and building stronger connections.

While having a supportive partner, friend, or family member is invaluable, the journey to better relationships starts with what you can do for yourself and those you care about. Together, you can create a foundation for mutual understanding and growth.

4.1 Masking ADHD

Living with ADHD often involves navigating a world designed for neurotypical individuals. One of the strategies many individuals with ADHD adopt to fit in is known as masking.

Masking refers to the conscious or unconscious effort to hide or suppress behaviors, traits, or symptoms associated with ADHD in order to fit societal norms or avoid judgment. This might mean forcing yourself to sit still when you naturally need to fidget, putting extra effort into staying organized to meet workplace expectations, or downplaying struggles with time management and focus.

At its core, masking is about adapting to a world that often misunderstands ADHD. While it can be a valuable tool in certain situations, relying on masking excessively can lead to burnout, emotional exhaustion, and other potential consequences and challenges.

Masking often stems from a desire to meet social expectations and avoid negative stereotypes associated with ADHD. Understanding what masking is, why it happens, and how to reduce its impact can empower you to live a more authentic and fulfilling life.

Social Pressures and the Desire to Conform

From a young age, individuals with ADHD may receive messages that their natural tendencies—such as restlessness, impulsivity, or difficulty focusing—are disruptive or unacceptable. Over time, this can create an internalized pressure to "blend in" by suppressing these traits.

In professional settings, for instance, someone with ADHD might feel compelled to appear hyper-organized and composed to avoid being labeled as unreliable. In social situations, they might stifle their natural enthusiasm or avoid conversations about their ADHD altogether to prevent being misunderstood.

Masking is often rooted in fear of rejection, judgment, or exclusion, making it a self-protective mechanism for navigating environments that lack understanding or support.

Consequences of Masking

While masking can help avoid uncomfortable situations in the short term, it often comes at a significant emotional and mental cost. Masking, over time, may cause distress and could even snowball into a breakdown if not handled and managed carefully.

Here's a list of other negative aspects of masking without proper guidance at an earlier stage:

- **Increased stress and anxiety:** Constantly monitoring and suppressing natural behaviors can be exhausting, leading to chronic stress and heightened anxiety. This mental strain can make it even harder to manage ADHD symptoms effectively, creating a vicious cycle.
- **A sense of isolation:** Masking often involves hiding a fundamental part of yourself, which can leave you feeling isolated and disconnected from others. If you're always

putting on a facade, it can be difficult to build genuine relationships where you feel truly understood and accepted.

- **Slow burn deterioration of mental health:** Over time, masking can erode self-esteem and contribute to feelings of inadequacy. It reinforces the idea that your true self isn't "good enough," which can lead to depression, emotional exhaustion, and a diminished sense of identity.

When your mental health becomes increasingly affected by masking almost every single day, especially when masking in itself is an unhealthy coping habit, the chances of you developing a mental illness—or comorbidity—become higher. The next best step is reducing the number of times you mask, and there are healthy ways to do so.

Strategies for Reducing Masking

While it's not always possible—or even necessary—to completely eliminate masking, adopting strategies that prioritize self-acceptance and authentic living can make a big difference.

Acknowledging your ADHD: The first step to reducing masking is acknowledging and accepting your ADHD as a part of who you are, not something to be hidden or fixed—it's about understanding that certain aspects of you need care and patience that are not only received from other people but from oneself.

This involves reframing ADHD traits as manageable differences rather than deficiencies or lack of normative traits. For instance, your need to fidget might help you focus, and your hyperfocus on topics of interest can be a strength—the differences you have from other people should never define your self-worth.

Authenticity and adaptation: While embracing your ADHD is important, it's also okay to adapt in ways that help you navigate certain situations more effectively. The goal isn't to mask completely but to find a balance that allows you to remain true to yourself while meeting the demands of your environment.

Reducing masking is about giving yourself permission to be authentic and recognizing that you don't need to conform to a one-size-fits-all standard. Surrounding yourself with people who understand and accept your ADHD can reduce the need to mask it—whether it's educating friends, family, or coworkers about ADHD or joining a support group, fostering environments where you feel safe to be yourself is key.

In professional settings, advocating for accommodations—like flexible work hours or a quiet workspace—can help you meet expectations without having to suppress your natural tendencies.

4.2 ADHD and Romantic Relationships

ADHD symptoms can influence romantic relationships in unique ways, but with awareness and proactive communication, these challenges can also become opportunities for growth and connection.

As mentioned previously in Chapter 2.4, Hyperfocus, a common ADHD trait, can lead to intense engagement in activities, projects, or interests, which may sometimes leave a partner feeling overlooked.

However, by setting boundaries and making time for shared moments, you can ensure your partner feels valued while still pursuing your passions.

Impulsivity, another hallmark of ADHD, may occasionally result in unfiltered comments or quick decisions. By practicing mindfulness and pausing to reflect before reacting, you can navigate these moments more thoughtfully, reducing potential misunderstandings.

Emotional sensitivity, while challenging at times, also brings depth and authenticity to relationships. By openly discussing emotional triggers and working together to manage them, couples can foster greater intimacy and mutual support.

With understanding, patience, and effort from both partners, ADHD can become a shared journey that strengthens the bond and enhances the relationship.

Here are some important factors to consider when you're in a romantic relationship:

Controlled Active Listening

If effective communication is the cornerstone of any healthy relationship, then it's even more critical when ADHD is part of the equation. Hyperfocus, while a unique strength, can lead to unintentional neglect of your partner's needs.

Practicing controlled active listening can help manage hyperfocus and ensure you remain attentive to your partner during conversations.

Controlled active listening involves being fully present and consciously redirecting your attention to your partner. Make eye contact, summarize what your partner says to ensure mutual understanding, and validate their feelings. For example, if your partner shares about a stressful day at work, respond with, "It sounds like you had a really tough day." This shows that you are listening to and valuing their experience.

Using "I" statements to express your feelings can also help maintain focus and manage hyperfocus. Instead of saying, "You never listen to me," try, "I feel hurt when I don't feel heard." This shifts the focus from blame to expressing your own experience, reducing defensiveness and promoting more constructive dialogue. Consciously practicing these techniques helps in balancing the intensity of hyperfocus with the necessity of being present in the moment, thereby fostering a healthier, more understanding relationship.

Scheduling Check-Ins

Scheduled check-ins and discussions are another effective strategy. Set aside regular times to talk about your relationship, discuss any issues, and celebrate successes. Doing this creates a structured space for communication, making it less likely that important conversations will be sidelined by daily distractions.

You could decide to have a weekly check-in every Sunday evening, where you both share your thoughts and feelings about the past week. This regular practice can help you stay connected and address issues before they escalate.

This is *especially* important when there's an important upcoming date that you need to remember.

The "Time-Out" Method

If conflicts arise, having strategies for constructive resolution is key—the "time-out" method can be particularly effective. Whenever emotions run high, take a break to cool down before continuing the conversation. Agree on a signal or phrase that indicates a need for a time-out, and, most importantly, *honor it*. This pause allows both of you to calm down and approach the issue with a clearer mind. For those with ADHD, this break can also serve as a moment to reset hyperfocus and redirect it toward resolving the conflict constructively.

Once you've had a chance to cool off, return to the discussion with a focus on collaborative problem-solving. Approach the conflict as a team, working together to find a solution that satisfies both parties—this might involve brainstorming different options and evaluating their pros and cons together.

Time, Love Language, Shared Activities

Strengthening the emotional bond in your relationship involves more than just managing conflicts.

Plan regular date nights to keep the romance alive. Set aside time to enjoy each other's company without the distractions of daily life—whether it's a fancy dinner out or a cozy night in with a movie, these moments of connection are essential.

Expressing appreciation and love is another powerful way to strengthen your bond. Simple acts like saying "thank you," leaving a sweet note, or even holding their hand (especially when it's cold or you're going through traffic) can go a long way in making your partner feel valued and loved.

Shared hobbies and activities can also bring you closer. Find something you both enjoy and make it a regular part of your routine—whether it's cooking, hiking, or painting. These shared experiences create lasting memories and deepen your connection.

Understanding how ADHD symptoms impact romantic relationships is the first step toward building healthier communication and stronger bonds. By practicing active listening, using "I" statements, scheduling regular check-ins, and employing constructive conflict resolution strategies, you can navigate the challenges and create a more fulfilling and loving relationship.

4.3 Cultivating Empathy with Family

ADHD can sometimes be misunderstood within families, even though it may have a genetic component or develop over time. While your loved ones might notice the symptoms, they may not always grasp the challenges that come with them.

Open and honest communication is key to fostering empathy and understanding. Sharing your experiences and providing resources about ADHD can help bridge the gap and create a supportive environment. By involving your family in the learning process, you give them the opportunity to understand the unique ways ADHD impacts your life. This mutual effort can strengthen relationships, cultivate empathy, and ensure that your family becomes a source of encouragement and support on your journey.

Open Family Discussions

Having open family discussions about ADHD can also be enlightening—creating a safe space where everyone can ask questions and express their feelings.

These conversations can potentially clear up misconceptions and foster a supportive environment. This type of conversation would require empathy, which doesn't come naturally to everyone, but it *can* be cultivated through specific exercises.

Role-playing scenarios are effective in helping family members understand your perspective. For example, switch roles and let them experience what it's like to manage ADHD symptoms while trying to complete daily tasks. This can be eye-opening and generate empathy.

Build an Empathy Map

Another way to cultivate empathy is through empathy mapping activities, which are another great tool. Create a map where family members can write down their thoughts, emotions, and experiences related to certain situations.

Then, compare these maps to see how perceptions differ. This exercise can bridge gaps in understanding and promote more empathetic interactions.

Set Up Boundaries

In talking about empathy, it's also important to set healthy boundaries and maintain a balanced relationship with family members. Clear communication of your needs is the first step; let your family know what you require to manage your ADHD effectively—whether it's needing quiet time to focus or requiring reminders for important tasks. Being upfront about your needs can prevent misunderstandings.

Respecting personal space is equally important. Make it clear when you need time alone to recharge and ensure that these boundaries are honored. Having this mutual respect can reduce friction and create a more harmonious living environment.

Family support strategies can make a significant difference in your daily life. From regular family meetings to discuss challenges and solutions, which can provide a structured time for everyone to share their experiences and brainstorm ways to support each other, to shared calendars for important dates, which can help keep everyone on the same page. Using a digital calendar that everyone can access to schedule family events, appointments, and deadlines is a shared responsibility, which can reduce the burden on you and ensure that nothing falls through the cracks.

Encouraging positive reinforcement is another effective strategy. Celebrate small achievements and acknowledge the efforts made to manage ADHD symptoms. Positive feedback can boost your self-esteem and motivate you to keep striving for improvement.

Educating your family about ADHD, engaging in empathy-building exercises, setting healthy boundaries, and implementing supportive strategies, can foster a more understanding and supportive environment at home. These efforts can lead to improved relationships, better communication, and a more harmonious family life.

4.4 Maintaining Your Social Circle

For many individuals with ADHD, making and maintaining friendships can feel like a balancing act, but it's entirely possible with the right strategies. Forgetfulness can sometimes create challenges, like unintentionally missing a meet-up or forgetting to return a call.

While this might lead to misunderstandings, simple tools such as setting reminders or using apps to stay organized can help you honor your commitments and show your friends how much you value them. Inconsistent communication patterns can also pose hurdles. You might experience periods of hyperfocus where conversations flow effortlessly, followed by quieter times when you need space. By being open with your friends about these patterns, you can foster understanding and reduce potential confusion.

Recognizing and addressing these dynamics proactively can help you nurture meaningful, lasting connections while embracing the unique qualities that make you a great friend.

Be Open About Your Struggles

Communicating your needs and limitations to friends is vital for managing these challenges. Begin by having an honest conversation about your ADHD—explain that your forgetfulness and communication gaps aren't a reflection of your feelings toward them but rather symptoms of your condition.

Being open about what you're struggling with can foster understanding and patience, and asking them for a bit of extra grace can give them the heads up that while you're working on improving these areas, you may need gentle reminders.

This straightforward approach can help set realistic expectations and reduce misunderstandings. It's also helpful to discuss specific ways they can support you, like sending a text reminder before a scheduled meetup.

Keep in Touch with Your Friends

Staying connected with friends requires intentional effort, especially when ADHD is in the mix. Regularly scheduled catch-ups can be a lifesaver. You can set a recurring time each week or month to connect with friends, whether it's a coffee date, a phone call, or a video chat. Building this routine can help ensure that you maintain those connections without relying solely on spontaneous interactions.

Using social media and messaging apps can also help bridge the gaps. Platforms like Facebook, Instagram, or WhatsApp allow you to stay updated on your friends' lives and send quick messages to check-in. These tools can make it easier to maintain communication, even during busy or overwhelming periods.

Share Experiences Together

Strengthening friendships goes beyond just staying in touch. Shared activities and interests can create deeper bonds. Find common hobbies or interests that you can enjoy together, like hiking, cooking, or playing board games. These shared experiences create lasting memories and provide a foundation for your friendship.

Thoughtful gestures and small surprises can also go a long way in showing your friends that you care. Simple acts like sending a funny meme, dropping off their favorite snack, or writing a heartfelt note can make them feel appreciated and loved. These gestures don't have to be grand or expensive; it's the thought that counts.

Open and honest communication is the bedrock of any strong friendship; make it a point to share your thoughts and feelings with your friends regularly. If you're struggling with something, *let them know*. If you're grateful for their support, *express it*. This transparency builds trust and deepens your connection. Similarly, encourage your friends to share their feelings and concerns with you—create a safe space where they can voice their thoughts without fear of judgment. This mutual openness can strengthen your friendship and create a more supportive and understanding relationship.

Navigating friendships with ADHD involves recognizing the challenges, communicating your needs, staying connected, and making an effort to strengthen your bonds. Forgetfulness and inconsistent communication patterns can strain friendships, but honest conversations about ADHD can foster understanding and patience.

Regularly scheduled catch-ups, using social media and messaging apps, shared activities, thoughtful gestures, and open communication can help you maintain and strengthen your friendships. By being intentional and proactive, you can build lasting and meaningful connections with your friends.

4.5 Tips for Reducing Social Anxiety

Many adults with ADHD may experience social anxiety, but there are ways to navigate these challenges and build confidence in social settings. The fear of judgment and rejection can sometimes feel overwhelming, leading to concerns about saying the wrong thing or being misunderstood.

However, focusing on your strengths, such as your creativity and ability to think on your feet, can help you approach social situations with a more positive mindset.

In busy environments, overstimulation can be a common issue, as noise, movement, and crowds might feel overwhelming. To manage this, consider strategies like finding quieter spaces for conversations, practicing mindfulness techniques to stay grounded, or setting boundaries to avoid sensory overload.

By recognizing your needs and using tools to support yourself, you can create more comfortable and enjoyable social experiences, allowing you to connect authentically with others.

Mentally Prepare

Mental preparation can make a significant difference when it comes to navigating social situations. Practicing conversation starters can help you feel more confident and something you can fall back on if you feel stuck, with a few different topics that you can bring up, like recent movies, books, or hobbies.

Visualization

Visualizing successful interactions is another effective technique. Before you go to an event, take a few minutes to imagine yourself having positive conversations and enjoying yourself. This mental rehearsal can reduce anxiety and boost your confidence.

Setting a time limit for social events can also be helpful. Decide in advance how long you'll stay. Knowing that you have an exit plan can make the situation feel more manageable and less overwhelming.

Breathe and Ground Yourself

During social interactions, coping strategies can especially help manage anxiety. When you start feeling anxious, you can try deep breathing exercises by taking slow, deep breaths to calm your mind and body.

Grounding techniques, like the 5-4-3-2-1 method, is a great method to anchor you in the present moment, and this can be done by identifying five things you can see, four things you can touch, three things you can hear, two things you can smell, and one thing you can taste.

Find a Buddy

The Buddy System also works great; bringing a supportive friend can provide a sense of security. Having someone you trust by your side can make social situations feel less intimidating and more enjoyable.

Reflection Journaling

Once a social event or interaction is done, reflecting on these afterward can help you learn and grow from each experience. You can do this by journaling about the experience, which is a great way to process your thoughts and feelings. Write down what went well and what you found challenging.

Reflecting on these can provide valuable insights for future interactions, focusing more on positive aspects instead of dwelling on what you think went wrong. Concentrate more on the moments you enjoyed and the connections you made. Then, plan for future improvements based on your reflections, and think about what you can do differently next time to feel more comfortable and confident. Navigating social situations with ADHD and social anxiety involves understanding how these conditions impact you and preparing accordingly.

Fear of judgment and overstimulation can make social interactions challenging, but practicing conversation starters, visualizing success, and setting time limits can help you feel more prepared. During interactions, coping strategies like deep breathing, grounding techniques, and bringing a supportive friend can manage anxiety.

Reflecting on your experiences through journaling, focusing on positives, and planning for improvements will help you grow more comfortable and confident in social settings. By integrating these techniques, you can enjoy social interactions more and build meaningful connections.

4.6 Workplace Relationships

In a business setting, the fast-paced environment and need for clear communication can present a unique set of hurdles and opportunities for growth and connection.

You may sometimes find it difficult to stay attentive during meetings or conversations, which could lead to missing details. However, by using tools such as note-taking, setting reminders, or seeking clarification when needed, you can minimize misunderstandings and enhance collaboration. Your enthusiasm and creative thinking can be valuable assets in team projects, though it's essential to find systems that help you track deadlines and requirements. Building trust with colleagues and supervisors can be achieved through consistent communication and follow-through on tasks.

Focusing on your strengths and seeking support when necessary will allow you to foster positive and productive workplace relationships, creating an environment where you and your team can thrive together.

Effective and Proactive Communication

Like with the other relationships we've discussed, effective communication is crucial for overcoming these challenges—though with added proactivity. In workplace communication, being clear and concise can make a significant difference.

When writing emails, get straight to the point and avoid unnecessary details. Use bullet points to break down complex information to make it easier for both you and the recipient to understand and respond. Regular status updates can also help keep everyone on the same page; send brief updates on your progress, even if there isn't much to report. This proactive communication shows your commitment and keeps your colleagues informed, reducing the risk of misunderstandings.

One-on-one meetings can be particularly effective for addressing any issues and clarifying expectations; these meetings can provide a focused environment where you can discuss tasks and receive feedback without the distractions of a group setting.

Networking and Support Systems

Building strong professional relationships involves more than just effective communication—networking within the workplace can open doors to new opportunities and create a support system. Attending company events, joining committees, or participating in group projects to meet new people and build connections can help you understand the workplace culture better and make you feel more integrated.

Actively participating in team-building activities is another great way to strengthen relationships. Such activities provide a relaxed environment where you can bond with colleagues outside of work tasks, fostering a sense of camaraderie and trust.

Other than your colleagues, seeking mentorship opportunities can also be incredibly beneficial. Find someone in your workplace whom you trust and admire, and ask if they'd be willing to mentor you. A mentor can offer valuable advice, provide feedback, and help you navigate the complexities of your job.

Workplace Accommodations

Workplace accommodations are another area to factor in to improve relationships and overall job performance. Flexible work hours can be a game changer, especially if you struggle with maintaining focus during traditional work hours. Talk to your supervisor about adjusting your schedule. Perhaps starting earlier or working later can help you find periods of peak productivity.

The use of organizational tools, which I mentioned in the third chapter, can help you stay on top of your responsibilities and meet deadlines, as these tools can reduce the cognitive load and make it easier to follow through on tasks.

Quiet workspaces are another valuable accommodation. If possible, request a workspace that minimizes distractions: A quieter environment can help you maintain focus and complete tasks more efficiently.

Understanding workplace dynamics and the specific challenges ADHD poses can help you develop strategies to improve communication and build stronger professional relationships. Miscommunications due to inattentiveness and difficulty following through on tasks are common issues, but clear and concise emails, regular status updates, and one-on-one meetings can mitigate these problems.

Building professional relationships through networking, team-building activities, and seeking mentorship opportunities can provide support and open doors to new opportunities.

Workplace accommodations like flexible work hours, organizational tools, and quiet workspaces can enhance your productivity and improve relationships with colleagues. The implementation of these strategies means that you can navigate the complexities of workplace relationships more effectively and create a much more supportive, understanding, and peaceful work environment.

4.7 Supporting Loved Ones with ADHD

If someone you care about has ADHD, your support can make an incredible difference in their life. Understanding ADHD isn't just about recognizing the condition—it's about seeing the world through their eyes and acknowledging the unique challenges they face daily.

This section is here to help you build stronger connections with your loved one by offering insights and strategies to provide meaningful support.

Educate Yourself to Build Empathy

The first step to supporting someone with ADHD is to educate yourself. ADHD isn't just about being distracted or hyperactive; it's a neurodevelopmental condition that impacts executive functions like organization, time management, and emotional regulation. By learning about ADHD, you can move beyond surface-level assumptions and better understand why your loved one might struggle with certain tasks.

For example, if they often forget important dates or misplace items, recognize that it's not a lack of care or effort. It's part of how their brain processes information. Reading books, attending workshops, or following reputable ADHD resources can help you develop empathy and gain tools to offer meaningful support.

Provide Emotional Support

Emotional support is at the heart of any strong relationship, especially when ADHD is involved. Often, individuals with ADHD feel misunderstood or judged for behaviors beyond their control. Your role is to create a safe space where they feel heard and valued.

- **Practice Active Listening:** When they share their struggles, give them your full attention. Avoid interrupting or rushing to provide solutions. Instead, acknowledge their feelings with phrases like, "That sounds really overwhelming. How can I help?" This simple act of listening can make them feel validated and supported.
- **Validate Their Experience:** Empathy goes a long way. Statements like, "It's okay to feel frustrated—it's a tough situation," show that you understand and accept their emotions without judgment.
- **Offer Encouragement:** Small affirmations can have a big impact. Phrases like, "You're doing your best, and that's enough," or "I'm proud of how hard you're working," can provide the motivation they need to keep going.

Offer Practical Support

Beyond emotional encouragement, practical support can significantly ease their daily challenges. ADHD often impacts organization, time management, and follow-through, and small gestures can make a big difference.

- **Help with Organization:** Assist in setting up tools like planners, digital calendars, or to-do lists that simplify their routines. For example, you might color-code a calendar to separate work, personal tasks, and relaxation time.

- **Provide Gentle Reminders:** Forgetfulness is a common ADHD symptom. A quick text about an appointment or a friendly nudge to prepare for an important meeting can be a lifesaver.
- **Collaborate on Routines:** Work together to create a balanced daily schedule that includes work, self-care, and leisure. Consistency helps manage ADHD symptoms and reduces stress.

Foster Independence

While your support is invaluable, it's also crucial to help your loved one build confidence and autonomy. Striking this balance requires patience and gradual steps.

- **Promote Self-Advocacy:** Encourage them to articulate their needs, whether it's asking for workplace accommodations or seeking therapy. Self-advocacy is a vital skill that empowers them to take control of their life.
- **Step Back Gradually:** Start by offering more hands-on assistance with tasks, but slowly reduce your involvement as they gain confidence and competence. This builds their independence without leaving them feeling overwhelmed.
- **Celebrate Their Wins:** Recognize and celebrate achievements, no matter how small. Acknowledge their effort with a simple "Great job completing that project" or "I'm proud of how you managed that situation." These moments of encouragement reinforce their progress and build self-esteem.

Be Patient and Adaptable

Supporting someone with ADHD is a journey, not a one-time effort. There will be setbacks, moments of frustration, and times when you might feel unsure of what to do. That's okay.

Remember, ADHD isn't a character flaw—it's a condition that requires understanding and adaptability. If one approach doesn't work, be willing to try something else. Your willingness to stick by them and adapt to their needs will create an environment where they feel supported, valued, and empowered to thrive. Educating yourself, offering emotional and practical support, and fostering independence can help you build a stronger relationship where your loved one can feel understood and appreciated.

Supporting someone with ADHD isn't about fixing them—it's about walking alongside them as they navigate their challenges and celebrate their successes. Together, you can create a partnership rooted in mutual respect and growth.

Make an Impact with Your Review

Help Someone on Their ADHD Journey

> *"The best way to predict the future is to create it."*

— Abraham Lincoln

By sharing your thoughts, you can inspire and support someone else who's navigating the complexities of ADHD.

My goal with ADHD Handbook is to provide actionable tools and hope to anyone seeking to understand and manage ADHD. But I can't reach everyone alone—your review makes all the difference.

Most people decide which book to read based on reviews. By leaving a review, you're helping others take a chance on learning strategies that could transform their lives. Your feedback could:

- Help a young adult realize they're not alone in their struggles.
- Encourage a parent to better understand their child.
- Motivate a teacher to create a more inclusive classroom.
- Support someone to embrace their ADHD as a strength, not a setback.

It takes just a moment to leave a review, but its impact can last a lifetime.

Thank you for making a difference and helping more people discover the tools they need to thrive.

With gratitude,
Kate Winslow

Chapter 5

ADHD and
Comorbidity Management

ADHD doesn't exist in isolation; it often intertwines with other mental health challenges, creating a complex landscape for those navigating its effects. This interconnectedness, known as comorbidity, refers to the occurrence of multiple conditions alongside ADHD, such as anxiety, depression, and mood disorders.

These overlapping conditions can amplify the challenges of managing ADHD, making it crucial to understand how they influence each other. By exploring these connections, we can uncover strategies to address not only ADHD but also the broader mental health picture, empowering individuals to thrive despite the complexities.

5.1 ADHD and Anxiety

You're lying in bed at night, staring at the ceiling, your mind racing with thoughts about tomorrow's deadlines, bills to pay, and that awkward conversation you had earlier. Your chest tightens, your heart pounds like a drum, and suddenly, it feels like the room is closing in. You try to take a deep breath, but it's like you can't get enough air.

Overthinking has escalated into an *anxiety attack.*

For many adults with ADHD, anxiety is a frequent companion. The link between ADHD and anxiety is complex but noteworthy—both conditions share overlapping symptoms, such as restlessness and difficulty concentrating—which can make it challenging to distinguish between the two.

While ADHD is primarily a neurodevelopmental disorder characterized by inattention, hyperactivity, and impulsivity, anxiety manifests as excessive worry, fear, and nervousness. The stress of managing ADHD symptoms can exacerbate anxiety levels, creating a vicious cycle where each condition feeds off the other. According to a study published in the Journal of Affective Disorders, more than half of adults with ADHD also experience anxiety disorders, highlighting the frequent coexistence of these conditions, and recognizing anxiety symptoms in the context of ADHD can be tricky.

Chronic worry and tension are hallmark signs of anxiety but can be masked by the restlessness common in ADHD. You might find yourself constantly on edge, worrying about things that others seem to brush off. Oftentimes, anxiety can also manifest itself physically through symptoms like headaches, stomachaches, and muscle tension, which are quite common.

These symptoms can be mistakenly attributed to other causes, delaying proper diagnosis and treatment. It's best to pay attention to these signs and consider them in the broader context of your ADHD diagnosis.

Managing Anxiety Symptoms

Coping with anxiety requires a multifaceted approach. One such approach is making use of Cognitive-Behavioral Techniques (CBT), which can be particularly effective since it focuses on identifying and altering negative thought patterns that contribute to anxiety.

Positive self-talk is a technique under CBT, so if you find yourself thinking, "I'll never get this done on time," this technique encourages you to challenge this thought and replace it with a more realistic one, like, "I can break this task into smaller steps and manage it." This shift in thinking can greatly reduce anxiety levels.

Progressive muscle relaxation (PMR) is another useful technique that involves tensing and then slowly releasing each muscle group in your body, starting from your toes and working up to your head. This method helps release physical tension and promotes a sense of calm—eventually, you will also find yourself subconsciously using this technique whenever your body tenses up due to stress or anxiety. Grounding exercises can usually provide immediate relief during an anxiety flare-up. One of the most effective techniques is the 5-4-3-2-1 method, which is structured like so:

1. 5 things you can **See**
2. 4 things you can **Touch**
3. 3 things you can **Hear**
4. 2 things you can **Smell**
5. 1 thing you can **Taste**

This grounding exercise shifts your focus away from anxious thoughts and anchors you in the present moment.

These methods can be helpful tools in your anxiety management toolkit, helping you regain control when anxiety threatens to overwhelm you.

5.2 ADHD and Depression

Most people with ADHD are more likely to develop depression compared to the general population, with these two conditions co-occurring.

With symptoms being extremely similar to each other, some adults don't get diagnosed with depression until much later, while others aren't diagnosed with ADHD and are diagnosed with depression instead. These two go hand-in-hand, making it complex and difficult to know which is which.

Let's start by understanding what depression is.

Depression is a mood disorder that is often identified by long-lasting feelings of sadness, hopelessness, and an increased lack of interest in activities. This affects how you think, feel, and handle daily activities. It can also cause insomnia, early-morning awakening despite sleeping so late, or even frequently oversleeping. Appetite may also change, and the person with depression can experience weight changes that range from mild to severe. Even the simplest tasks feel impossible.

Next, let's understand how chronic ADHD works, especially *with* depression, to shed light on the similarities with depression.

Chronic ADHD symptoms can actively wear you down, leading to persistent feelings of inadequacy and frustration. When you're constantly struggling to keep up, it's easy to fall into a pattern of hopelessness. Untreated ADHD can exacerbate these feelings as the daily battles with organization, focus, and impulsivity accumulate into a sense of despair. The impact on your mood can be profound, making it difficult to find joy in activities you once loved.

Noticing signs of depression in the context of ADHD can be challenging, but it's extremely crucial. Seemingly never-ending sadness and a loss of interest in activities are key indicators. You might find that hobbies you once enjoyed no longer bring you pleasure or that your motivation to engage with loved ones has waned.

Fluctuations in appetite and sleep patterns are also common. Some people may overeat as a way to cope, while others lose their appetite altogether. Similarly, sleep can become disrupted; you might struggle with insomnia or find yourself sleeping excessively. Such changes can be subtle and gradual, making them easy to miss, especially when ADHD symptoms are already making daily life feel chaotic.

Managing depression alongside ADHD requires a multifaceted approach—establishing a daily routine can bring about a sense of structure and predictability, which is often comforting when you're feeling low. Many of these techniques may be hard to do for now, but what matters is that you didn't just try; you *did* these approaches. Do your best to wake up and go to bed at the same time each day, and include activities that promote physical and mental well-being. Taking part in regular physical activities, such as light or heavy exercises, is an effective strategy to improve mood by releasing endorphins—the body's natural feel-good chemicals.

Even a short walk can make a difference. Setting small, achievable goals is also important, and it's important that you're aware that minor tasks can feel overwhelming. Make use of the chunking method; break your day into manageable chunks and reinforce achieved tasks by celebrating them. This can help build momentum and combat the inertia that often accompanies depression. It's not an overnight approach, but it can be a great start. Knowing when to seek professional help is also just as important. If you experience persistent symptoms, it's time to consult a healthcare provider. This includes chronic sadness, a lack of interest in life, or significant changes in sleep and appetite.

Thoughts of self-harm or suicide are particularly urgent and require immediate attention. Professional help can come in various forms. Therapy, such as CBT, has proven effective for many people. A therapist can help you set up coping strategies tailored to your specific needs. Balancing ADHD and depression is a delicate process, but it's manageable with the right strategies and support.   It's crucial to know when to approach a professional for help and understand your treatment options to cope with both conditions effectively.

5.3 ADHD and Autism

ADHD and autism aren't the same thing, even if both can sometimes have similar traits—even co-occurring with one another in some individuals. But they're both different in the way that they function.

Where those with ADHD can mostly be more associated with difficulties in placing their focus on one thing at a time or even behaving impulsively, those with ASD (Autism Spectrum

Disorder) have a broader range of developmental issues, which includes communication and or social interaction.

Those with ASD also have more restricted or repetitive behaviors—having a strong preference for routines as well. Despite their differences, there are similarities between these two neurodivergent conditions, which can make the diagnosis and treatment complex.

Complex Co-Occurrence of ADHD and ASD

The combined symptoms can amplify difficulties when ADHD and ASD are simultaneously present within an individual.

- **Executive Function Difficulties:** Both ADHD and ASD individuals may find it challenging to properly manage executive functions, such as planning, organization, and time management.
- **Attention Challenges:** Difficulty maintaining attention and focus can be present in both conditions, although the underlying reasons might differ.
- **Sensory Sensitivities:** Both may experience heightened sensitivities to sensory stimuli like sounds, lights, textures, and smells.
- **Social Interaction Difficulties:** Challenges in social interactions, such as understanding social cues or forming and maintaining relationships, can occur in both.
- **Emotional Regulation:** Both conditions can involve difficulties with managing emotions, leading to heightened reactions or outbursts.
- **Routine and Structure:** A preference for routine and structure can be seen in both, although in ASD, it tends to be more pronounced and rigid.

Overall, the co-occurrence of ADHD and ASD requires a more fine-tuned and comprehensive approach to support and intervention, as the interplay of these conditions can heavily influence daily functioning and quality of life.

Research into the ADHD-ASD Overlap

Thankfully, there has been recent research that has shed new light on the overlap and distinctions between ADHD and ASD and offers a fresh perspective on these neurodevelopmental disorders. The study, titled *"Unraveling the Spectrum: Overlap, Distinctions, and Nuances of ADHD and ASD in Children,"* explores the clinical presentation of similarities and differences in ADHD and ASD, focusing on deficits in executive function, social function, and emotional intelligence.

The study highlights how both ADHD and ASD can exacerbate deficiencies in these areas, presenting significant diagnostic challenges. Individuals with these conditions often exhibit similar behaviors and struggle with navigating their environments. The research underscores the importance of refining diagnostic methods and treatments to improve outcomes for those affected by these disorders.

5.4 ADHD and Sensory Processing

Sensory processing refers to the brain's ability to interpret and respond to sensory information, such as sounds, sights, smells, textures, and movement.

For about 60-69% of individuals with ADHD—or those with other neurological or psychological conditions regardless of whether it is co-occurring *with or without* ASD—this process can sometimes be heightened or altered, which leads to either sensory sensitivities or sensory-seeking behaviors.

SPD and Sensory Sensitivities

Sensory Processing Disorder (SPD) is often seen in conditions such as ASD and ADHD. It encompasses a range of sensory processing issues where the brain may find it challenging to receive and respond to sensory input, including both hypersensitivity and hyposensitivity.

As this disorder can overlap with ADHD, it makes it challenging to differentiate and diagnose. Sensory sensitivity, on the other hand, is a component of other conditions, *including* SPD, and is more specific to heightened awareness or reactivity to certain stimuli.

Sensory-Seeking Behaviors

When there is a need for additional sensory input, one may seek it by engaging in actions that usually involve movement and touching certain objects to feel balanced or focused. This behavior is often seen in individuals with ADHD and may include actions like:

- **Fidgeting**: Tapping, bouncing legs, or playing with small objects.
- **Exploring Textures**: Touching soft fabrics, rough surfaces, or other tactile experiences.
- **Craving Movement**: Pacing, swinging arms, hopping, or engaging in high-energy activities.

Without proper understanding and management, these sensory-seeking behaviors can become overwhelming and disruptive. It's best to recognize and address these needs to *maintain balance* instead of *feeling balanced*, preventing them from negatively impacting daily life.

Sensory Overload

When one is exposed to an environment with excessive sensory input, the brain can become overwhelmed, resulting in a sensory overload.

This neurological condition can significantly impact an individual's ability to function and process information effectively, and it's often associated with certain environments and stimuli that can become unbearable to process. The severity of symptoms could determine how much more sensitive and vulnerable your senses could become.

Unfortunately, some people faced with a simultaneous sensory dump may freeze or get 'stuck' (i.e., zoning out or disassociating) since the brain can't prioritize which sensory information it needs to focus on. There are several external stimuli that could trigger a sensory overload, with the more common triggers usually being those that could intensify and easily overcome your senses.

Here are some of the more common triggers with their usual sources:

- **Loud Noises**: crowded spaces, alarms, extremely loud music, or overlapping conversations.
- **Bright Lights:** fluorescent lights, sunlight, multiple car headlights at night, or screen glare.
- **Crowded Environments**: Busy malls, tight public transport, school areas, or social gatherings.

Once a person with ADHD is exposed to certain triggers and begins experiencing sensory overload, they may experience various symptoms that can cause them to either freeze or, in severe cases, have a meltdown.

Symptoms, though varying, will often include:

- **Physical Symptoms**: Headaches, tension, or a racing heart.
- **Emotional Reactions**: Anxiety, irritability, or feelings of being overwhelmed.
- **Cognitive Struggles**: Difficulty focusing, zoning out, or wanting to escape the situation.

If left unchecked, these symptoms can intensify if you or the person with you is exposed to such external stimuli—leading to even more extreme episodes.

Once you notice that you, or someone close to you, seems to be experiencing sensory overload, it's crucial to do the following:

- **Find a Quiet Space**: Move to a quieter, less stimulating environment to reduce the intensity of sensory input.
- **Deep Breathing**: Take slow, deep breaths to help calm your nervous system.
- **Grounding Techniques**: Do grounding exercises, such as focusing on the physical sensations of touching a textured object, counting backwards, or describing your surroundings in detail.
- **Close Your Eyes**: Temporarily closing your eyes can help reduce visual input and give your brain a break.
- **Use Noise-Canceling Headphones**: If you're sensitive to sound, noise-canceling headphones can help block out overwhelming noises.

- **Weighted Blanket or Vest**: Using a weighted blanket or vest can provide comforting pressure and help calm your body.

Positive Outlets for Sensory Seeking

Utilizing sensory-seeking tendencies in constructive ways can improve focus and reduce frustration.

Consider these activities:

- **Fidget Toys**: Items like stress balls, spinners, or putty provide sensory stimulation without being disruptive.
- **Sensory Bins**: Fill a bin with sand, rice, or small objects to explore textures and calm the mind.
- **Physical Exercise**: Activities like yoga, jumping on a trampoline, or going for a run can fulfill the need for movement while enhancing overall well-being.

By understanding sensory processing in ADHD, you can create strategies to navigate both sensory sensitivities and sensory-seeking behaviors.

Chapter 6

Emotional Resilience
and Self-Management

Living with ADHD comes with its own set of challenges, from battling procrastination to managing emotional overwhelm. These hurdles, while significant, are not insurmountable. By adopting the right coping mechanisms, you can rework these challenges into opportunities for growth and self-discovery.

This chapter delves into actionable strategies designed to empower you in your ADHD journey. From creating structured routines to practicing mindfulness and seeking external support, you'll learn how to build habits that foster focus, confidence, and resilience.

Understanding your unique needs and tailoring these strategies to fit your lifestyle is a keystone to bettering yourself and your emotional resilience. By equipping yourself with personalized tools and approaches, you'll not only manage the symptoms of ADHD but also thrive, enhancing your overall well-being and unlocking your full potential.

6.1 Coping Mechanisms

Coping mechanisms are the strategies you use to adapt to stress, emotions, or difficult situations. For those with ADHD, these can help manage common challenges like procrastination, impulsivity, and emotional overwhelm.

When done right, effective coping mechanisms can bring clarity to chaotic situations, improve focus, and build confidence. However, the *wrong* habits, even if they feel comforting at the moment, can worsen such challenges over time. That's why understanding and choosing the right strategies is essential.

Negative Coping Strategies

First, when dealing with a difficult emotion or episode, it's important to know when to spot and avoid unhealthy coping mechanisms. Again, these unhealthy coping strategies may offer temporary relief—but can often lead to long-term harm or abuse towards oneself or even others.

Some of these harmful coping strategies are:

- **Avoidance**: Procrastination is a common challenge for individuals with ADHD, but it often leads to heightened anxiety as deadlines loom. Avoidance can create a vicious cycle, making tasks feel even more daunting over time.
- **Self-Medication**: While substances like caffeine, alcohol, or even recreational drugs may seem like quick fixes to boost focus or relax, they often backfire, exacerbating symptoms and creating dependency.
- **Overworking**: Many adults with ADHD fall into the trap of overworking to compensate for perceived shortcomings. While this may feel productive at first, it can lead to burnout, exhaustion, and a decline in physical and mental health.

Positive Coping Strategies

Next, we identify the healthy coping mechanisms that can empower you in managing ADHD symptoms, as well as create a more balanced life.

Here are some proven strategies:

- **Routine Building**: Routines provide structure and predictability, which are vital for those with ADHD. A consistent routine helps reduce decision fatigue and gives your day a clear direction.
- **Mindfulness Practices**: Practicing mindfulness can help calm the racing thoughts that often accompany ADHD.
- **Physical Exercise**: Exercising is another healthy way to manage ADHD symptoms, which can be done by doing activities you enjoy—which will release endorphins, improve mood, and sharpen focus.
- **Seeking Support**: You don't have to manage ADHD alone. Therapy, support groups, or even a trusted friend can provide encouragement and fresh perspectives. Talking openly with family members about your challenges and needs can strengthen relationships and foster understanding.

Developing Healthy Coping Mechanisms

The path to effective coping begins with self-awareness and a commitment to growth.

- **Self-Awareness**: Understanding your triggers is the first step to managing them. Pay attention to patterns—are you more distracted after long meetings or when you're feeling overwhelmed? Journaling can help identify these triggers.
- **Personalizing Strategies**: Not all coping mechanisms work for everyone. Experiment with different approaches to find

what resonates with you. For instance, some might thrive with a rigid schedule, while others prefer a more flexible routine.

- **Building Resilience**: Life with ADHD is filled with ups and downs, but resilience helps you bounce back. Celebrate small victories and focus more on making progress rather than seeking perfect results. By cultivating self-compassion, you'll strengthen your ability to adapt and grow, no matter the challenges.

Reaching Out to Groups and Sharing Experiences

Expanding more into seeking support; finding your community can seem a bit more difficult than it should be, but there are several easy pathways to explore.

Local support groups are a great place to start. These groups offer face-to-face interactions where you can share your experiences and learn from others. You can always check community centers or local health organizations for meeting schedules with these support groups.

Social media groups and online forums provide another avenue for connection. Platforms like *Reddit*, *Facebook*, and specialized ADHD forums are bustling with activity and support; these virtual communities offer flexibility, allowing you to engage at your own pace and comfort level. Interacting with these communities may also be a bit more comforting if you prefer to keep yourself anonymous.

ADHD organizations and advocacy groups offer a plethora of resources and opportunities to connect with others. These organizations often host events, webinars, and forums where you can meet individuals who have similar views, as well as learn from experts.

6.2 Building Resilience Against Stress

Living with ADHD often means navigating a landscape filled with stress; the difficulty in managing daily responsibilities can make simple tasks feel like monumental challenges.

Whether it's forgetting an important meeting or losing track of time, these daily hurdles can accumulate, creating a constant undercurrent of stress—sensitivity to environmental stimuli further compounds this issue—with loud noises, bright lights, or even the chatter of a busy office which can overwhelm your senses, making it harder to concentrate and complete tasks.

This heightened sensitivity makes it crucial to find effective stress-reduction techniques tailored to your needs.

Breathe Slowly and Deeply

One effective way to reduce stress is through deep breathing exercises, which can be done just about and don't require any special equipment. Find a quiet spot, sit comfortably, and take deep breaths in and out, in through your nose and out through your mouth. Follow the rhythm of your breath, allowing it to slow down your heart rate and calm your mind. If there's no quiet spot and if you can't sit, don't worry—breathing exercises can still be done standing up, and if you have headphones or earplugs—something to muffle the noise—then that can work to create a quiet domain for yourself.

Reduce Your Workload

Another technique is time management and delegation. Knowing when to delegate tasks can significantly reduce your workload and stress levels. Make a list of your daily responsibilities and check which tasks can be delegated to others.

Doing these will not only lighten your load, but also allow you to focus more on demanding, high-priority tasks that require your attention.

Try Creative Hobbies

Creative outlets like art or music can serve as excellent stress relievers. Engaging in creative activities allows your mind to shift focus from stressors to something enjoyable and fulfilling; whether it's by painting, playing an instrument, or writing, all of these activities can provide a mental break, helping you return to your tasks with a more refreshed mind and perspective.

Adding these techniques into your daily routine can make a significant difference in managing stress levels—building resilience to stress involves developing a growth mindset, where instead of viewing challenges as obstacles, you see them more as opportunities.

Rationally Approach Problems

Strengthening problem-solving skills is another crucial aspect of building resilience. When faced with a stressful situation, break it down into smaller, manageable parts. Identify the root cause of the problem and brainstorm potential solutions. This methodical approach can make even the most daunting problems seem more manageable.

Live a Healthier Lifestyle

With ADHD, it can become difficult to commit to self-care practices as a daily routine for long-term stress management. However, it can be extremely beneficial in the long run, not just for stress management but for your overall quality of life.

Engaging in regular physical activity, especially aiming for at least 30 minutes of moderate exercise, such as walking, cycling, or yoga, most days of the week can help release endorphins while keeping you in shape and active.

Balanced nutrition is equally important; with a diet that is rich in fruits, vegetables, lean proteins, and whole grains, you can receive the necessary nutrients your body needs to function optimally. It's also best to avoid consuming an excess of caffeine and sugar as much as possible since these can contribute to anxiety and stress. If you're struggling to establish a healthier lifestyle, you can check *Chapter 7* of this book, which focuses more on *Lifestyle Changes.*

Get Proper Sleep

Adequate rest and relaxation are vital for stress management; make sure you get about 7-9 hours of quality sleep each night. You can set up a bedtime routine that includes wind-down activities like reading or taking a warm bath, as this signals your body that it's time to relax and prepare for sleep. During the day, take short breaks to rest and recharge.

Even a brief 5-minute break can help clear your mind and improve focus. Remember, self-care isn't selfish; it's a necessity for maintaining your mental and physical health.

Take a moment to try this quick stress-reduction exercise. Find a quiet spot where you won't be disturbed. Sit or lie down comfortably. Close your eyes and take a deep breath in through your nose, counting to four. Hold your breath and count to four, then exhale slowly through your mouth while counting to four again. Repeat this process five times. Notice how your body feels more relaxed and your mind calmer. This simple exercise can be especially useful whenever you feel overwhelmed or stressed.

If you're having difficulty winding down, which is quite common, you're not alone. Some with ADHD can't easily transition from the day's activities to a restful state. Irregular sleep patterns often follow, making it hard to maintain a consistent sleep schedule. You might find yourself wide awake at midnight and struggling to get out of bed in the morning. These sleep issues are more than just an inconvenience; they can exacerbate ADHD symptoms and affect your overall health.

First, create a sleep-friendly environment to improve your rest. Start by reducing noise and light in your bedroom. Use blackout curtains to limit or completely block external light, and for drowning out disruptive sounds, consider using a white noise machine or app.

If you don't have comfortable bedding, try to find one that is suited to your personal tastes—a softer bedding is advisable. Next, invest in a mattress and pillows that support your sleep posture and preferences. And finally, keep your bedroom temperature cool, around 60–67°F (15–19°C), to create an optimal sleeping environment. These changes can help signal to your brain that it's time to wind down and prepare for rest.

Then, establish a consistent bedtime routine that sets the stage for better sleep. You can do this by laying out a regular sleep schedule: Go to bed and try to consistently wake up at the same time every day, especially on weekends. Doing this can help regulate your internal clock and can even make falling asleep easier. You can also try adding relaxation techniques before bed to signal to your body that it's time to unwind.

Limiting screen time before sleep is essential, as the blue light from screens can interrupt your body's melatonin production; turning off electronic devices about an hour before bedtime can help prepare you for sleep. Following these steps can help create a calming pre-sleep ritual that allows a seamless transition to sleep.

Use this checklist to assess and improve your sleep hygiene:

- Reduce noise and light in your bedroom.
- Invest in comfortable bedding and maintain a cool room temperature.
- Set a regular sleep schedule and stick to it every day, even on weekends.
- Incorporate relaxation techniques like reading or meditation before bed.
- Limit screen time at least an hour before bedtime.
- If none of these work, it might be time to consult with a sleep specialist in case of a sleep disorder.

Review this checklist regularly to ensure you're maintaining habits that promote better sleep.

Making these adjustments can create a more conducive environment for rest, helping you manage ADHD symptoms more effectively.

6.3 Developing a Positive Mindset

When life throws curveballs at someone with ADHD, it can sometimes feel like an entire boulder of disappointment.

However, resilience is your ability to bounce back from setbacks, which is an important trait to develop, *especially* when you have ADHD. Given how life can throw many difficult challenges, a well-built resilience will allow you to grow a more positive outlook despite the tough hurdles. It means not giving up when things go wrong and instead finding ways to cope and move forward. It's like a mental muscle that gets stronger each time it's used.

By training and building this muscle, you allow yourself to navigate life's ups and downs without getting completely derailed.

Kind Self-Talk

Developing a resilient mindset starts with practicing positive self-talk. Negative thoughts can be a constant companion, especially when dealing with ADHD. You miss an appointment or forget an important task, and the self-criticism begins. Instead of berating yourself, try flipping the script and reminding yourself of your strengths and past successes.

Positive self-talk can shift your perspective, making setbacks feel more like temporary inconveniences than insurmountable obstacles.

Personal Growth Mindset

Embracing a growth mindset is another powerful strategy. This means viewing life's hurdles and challenges as a chance to learn and grow rather than *just* seeing them as failures.

When you encounter a setback, you *can* feel hurt, but you have to ask yourself what you can learn from the experience.

You can give yourself time to grieve over a failure, but this shift in thinking can transform obstacles into valuable lessons rather than a moment to continuously dwell on.

Learn from Mistakes

Learning from failures and setbacks is the very foundation of resilience. Each setback offers a chance to gain insight and improve. Reflect on what went wrong, but also on what went right. Identify the factors within your control and those outside it.

This reflection helps you develop better strategies for the future. A good example of this would be when you missed a deadline. Analyze *why* it happened. Was it a lack of planning, or were there unforeseen circumstances? Use this information to fine-tune your approach next time.

Reflective Resilience-Building Exercises

Resilience-building exercises can strengthen your ability to cope with challenges. Writing about past challenges and how you overcame them can be incredibly empowering—it reminds you of your capacity to handle difficulties and reinforces your resilience.

Participating in semi-active activities like yoga or meditation can also enhance resilience. These practices teach you to stay present, manage stress, and maintain emotional balance. Keeping a gratitude journal is another effective exercise.

Each day, write down a few things you're grateful for. This practice shifts your focus from what's going wrong to what's going right, fostering a more positive outlook.

Connect with Supportive Peers

Support systems, where you connect with friends and family, can provide a safety net and help you build resilience. These relationships offer emotional support, advice, and encouragement when you need it most. Joining support groups, either in person or online, can help you feel a sense of belonging and mutual empathy. Knowing that you're not alone in your struggles can be comforting. And seeking professional counseling or coaching is another option—a therapist or coach can provide targeted strategies to build resilience and help you navigate challenges more effectively.

Positive self-talk, a growth mindset, and learning from setbacks are powerful tools for increased resilience. Other resilience-building exercises like writing, yoga, and keeping a gratitude journal can further strengthen your ability to bounce back. Support systems, both personal and professional, provide the foundation you need to maintain this resilience. Each of these elements contributes to a more robust, adaptable, and positive approach to life's inevitable challenges.

6.4 Self-Worth Exercises

Living with ADHD comes with unique challenges, often compounded by misunderstandings. Missed deadlines or forgotten tasks are frequently misjudged as laziness rather than symptoms of a legitimate condition, leading to feelings of judgment, isolation, and frustration.

These unfair misconceptions can deeply affect self-perception, fueling comparisons with others and fostering a distorted self-image where ADHD feels like a limitation rather than just one aspect of who you are.

Personally, you may feel like an underachiever, struggling to meet expectations from family or friends. Professionally, finding a career that suits your strengths might seem daunting, resulting in instability or frequent job changes.

However, these challenges don't have to define you, and practicing self-compassion can break this cycle. Treat yourself by giving yourself the same kindness you'd offer a friend; instead of just labeling yourself as a failure, try reframing mistakes as opportunities to learn: "What can I learn from this to prevent this from happening again? How can I break away from my own cycle?"

Self-care is another vital part of self-compassion. Activities that foster your mental and emotional health, like enjoying a hobby, taking a walk, or practicing mindfulness, are one of the many ways to engage in self-care. Accept yourself as you are—flaws and all—and focus on the present without judgment.

Forgiveness is also key; let go of past mistakes, not to excuse them but to acknowledge and grow from them. Writing a compassionate response to a past error, such as, "I did my best with what I knew then, and I'm still learning," can help.

Building a compassionate inner voice requires practice but is transformative. Replace negative thoughts like, "I'm terrible at this," with affirmations like, "I'm learning and improving." Keep a journal of accomplishments to shift your focus to strengths rather than shortcomings.

Requesting feedback from trusted friends or mentors can also provide valuable perspective and reinforce positive qualities.

Start each day with empowering thoughts. Replace self-doubt with affirmations like, "I'm capable, and I'll learn from whatever comes my way." Treat yourself with kindness to foster resilience and growth. By forgiving yourself and embracing self-compassion, you create a supportive foundation for navigating the challenges of ADHD with confidence and grace.

You can shape a fulfilling life by building strategies to leverage your strengths and overcome obstacles. Empowering yourself with practical solutions is about acknowledging difficulties and actively working to overcome them.

With persistence, acknowledgment, and support from yourself, you don't have to see yourself as just being defined by your condition. You are loved, and if you are loved, that means you yourself are not voided of love *for* yourself and are fully capable of doing so. Allowing self-love will become your strength, a stronger foundation for self-esteem, and a strong sense of self-worth.

When these issues are left unchecked for a very long time, in some scenarios, it may even result in the development of the comorbidities mentioned within this chapter. It can become quite difficult to cope with but *not* impossible to solve.

6.5 More Mindfulness Techniques

At this point in the book, you may now be a bit more familiar with mindfulness, which is the practice of being fully present in the moment. This can significantly benefit individuals with ADHD. Mindfulness has been shown to improve focus and attention. By training your mind to stay present, you can reduce the mental clutter that often distracts you. This deepened focus can make it easier to complete tasks and stay on track.

One of the other benefits of mindfulness is its ability to reduce impulsivity and stress. When you're mindful, you're more aware of your thoughts and actions, which allows you to pause before reacting impulsively. This pause can be crucial in preventing hasty decisions that you might later regret. This also helps in managing stress by promoting a sense of calm and relaxation. When you're less stressed, your ADHD symptoms can become more manageable, creating a positive feedback loop that enhances your overall well-being.

Incorporating mindfulness into your regular routine doesn't have to be complicated, and you can start through mindful eating. Focus on your food's flavors, textures, and smells. Chew slowly and savor each bite. This practice not only enhances your eating experience but also helps you stay present.

Mindful walking is another easy way to integrate mindfulness. As you walk, pay close attention to the sensations you feel under your feet: the ground, the steady sequence and beat of each of your own steps, and slowly lead it up to the sights and sounds around you. This simple grounding exercise can turn a mundane activity into a calming experience.

There are several other mindfulness exercises that can be particularly effective for individuals with ADHD.

Body Scan Meditation

One such exercise is body scan meditation. This involves lying down or sitting in any position you find comfortable and focusing your attention on different parts of your body—starting from your toes and moving up to your head.

As you focus on each part, notice any sensations or tension and consciously relax those areas. This practice helps improve your mind-body connection and promotes relaxation.

Mindful Breathing

Mindful breathing is another powerful technique. Find a quiet space, sit comfortably, and focus on your breath. Then, feel the sensation of air entering and leaving your nostrils, or maybe even the rise and fall of your chest—or both. If your attention begins to waver, gently bring it back to your breath. This simple exercise can be done wherever you go and serves as a quick way to center and ground yourself when you're feeling overwhelmed.

Guided Imagery

Guided imagery is another beneficial mindfulness technique that involves imagining a serene scene, such as a beach or a forest, and immersing yourself in that environment. Imagine the sounds, smells, and sensations you would experience. Guided imagery can be particularly helpful before bed or during breaks, providing a mental escape that refreshes your mind.

Short Breaks

Short mindfulness breaks during the day can also be incredibly effective. Take a few minutes between tasks to close your eyes and focus on your breath or do a quick body scan. These mini breaks can help reset your mind and improve your focus for the next task.

Technology offers various tools to support your mindfulness practice. Guided meditation apps are tailored to different needs, from stress reduction to improved focus, through short, manageable sessions that can conveniently fit into your busy schedule.

Sleep apps are known for providing relaxation and sleep-focused content, as well as featuring guided meditations, sleep stories, and calming music for unwinding.

Some relaxation apps will offer even more meditation options that also include timed meditations while also including a community feature, allowing you to connect with others on a similar path.

Incorporating these mindfulness practices and tools into your daily routine can make a big difference in managing ADHD symptoms. By improving focus, reducing impulsivity, and alleviating stress, mindfulness can provide a much-needed anchor in a world that often feels overwhelming.

Chapter 7

Strength-Based Approaches for ADHD

ADHD comes with its challenges, but it also brings unique strengths that, when harnessed effectively, can lead to personal growth and fulfillment. In this chapter, we'll explore how to embrace and build upon these natural abilities, transforming perceived limitations into opportunities for success.

We'll delve into the power of hyperfocus, a tool that, when directed wisely, can unlock extraordinary productivity. Creativity and diffused thinking, often associated with ADHD, can spark innovative solutions and fresh ideas. Additionally, we'll examine emotional intelligence and problem-solving skills, essential traits that allow you to navigate relationships and challenges with empathy and resilience.

You'll also discover how leadership qualities, such as adaptability and vision, can emerge from your unique ADHD perspective. Finally, by recognizing and celebrating your strengths, you'll learn to reframe your ADHD as an asset rather than a setback, paving the way for a life that aligns with your potential and passions.

7.1 Advantageous Use of Hyperfocus

Picture this: you're deeply immersed in a project, completely absorbed in the task at hand. Hours slip by unnoticed—dinner is forgotten, messages go unread, and suddenly, dawn breaks through your window. That said, hyperfocus can definitely be a double-edged sword for adults with ADHD.

On one hand, hyperfocus allows you to channel extraordinary productivity and delve into tasks with remarkable precision. It's as if the world narrows to just you and your work, enabling you to immerse yourself so deeply that everything else fades away.

This can be particularly powerful when applied to hobbies or familiar tasks where muscle memory and creativity flow seamlessly.

However, this intense concentration can also have its downsides. It's easy to lose track of time, neglect other responsibilities, or feel out of balance when hyperfocus takes over. The challenge lies in harnessing this ability without letting it disrupt other important aspects of your life. By learning to balance hyperfocus with awareness and prioritization, you can transform it into one of your greatest assets.

Understanding what triggers your hyperfocus in order to harness it productively.

Hyperfocus often kicks in when you're engaged in tasks that are intrinsically interesting or align with your passions. Think about the projects that make you lose track of time. Maybe it's a creative endeavor like painting, a technical task like coding, or even a simple hobby like gardening—these activities captivate your attention because they resonate with your interests and strengths.

Identifying these triggers can help you strategically plan your work around them, ensuring you can tap into hyperfocus when needed.

Leveraging hyperfocus for productivity involves setting specific goals for your focus sessions. Before diving into a task, outline what you aim to achieve; break the task into smaller, manageable goals. For example, if you're writing a report, set a goal to complete the introduction in one session, followed by the body and conclusion in subsequent sessions. This approach not only makes the task less overwhelming but also provides a clear roadmap to follow.

Creating an optimal work environment is equally crucial. Find a quiet space free from distractions, and gather all the materials you need beforehand. This way, you can dive into your work without interruptions.

Scheduling hyperfocus sessions during peak productivity times can further enhance your efficiency. Each and every individual has their own specific peak-productivity hours of the day when they feel the most alert and focused. Identify these times and reserve them for tasks that require deep concentration. For some, early mornings might be ideal, while others might find late evenings more conducive to hyperfocus.

Experiment with different times to discover what works best for you. Once you align your work schedule with your natural rhythms, you can maximize the benefits of hyperfocus. However, balancing hyperfocus with other responsibilities is essential to avoid neglecting important duties.

To do this, set timers or alarms to help you take breaks and shift your focus when needed. You can effectively try this by using a timer to work in 90-minute intervals, followed by a 15-minute break. During these breaks, step away from your work and stretch or grab a snack. Short pauses like these can refresh your mind and prevent burnout. It's also important to prioritize tasks to ensure that your hyperfocus sessions are directed toward high-impact activities.

Create a daily or weekly task list, ranking items by importance and urgency. This way, you can allocate your hyperfocus to tasks that truly matter.

Consider using a tool like the Eisenhower Matrix to categorize your tasks. This matrix helps you distinguish between urgent and important tasks, ensuring that you focus on what's most critical; if you have a pressing work deadline and a personal project you're passionate about, prioritize the work task first.

Once it's completed, you can reward yourself by diving into your personal project.

This balanced approach allows you to harness the power of hyperfocus without letting other responsibilities fall by the wayside.

Reflection Exercise: Identifying Your Hyperfocus Triggers

Take a moment to reflect on your past experiences with hyperfocus. Think about the tasks or activities that have captured your undivided attention.

Use the following questions to guide your reflection:

1. What tasks or activities make you lose track of time?
2. What common elements do these tasks share (e.g., creativity, problem-solving, physical activity)?
3. How do these tasks align with your interests and passions?
4. When during the day do you feel most focused and alert?

Write down your answers and look for patterns. This exercise can provide valuable insights into your hyperfocus triggers, helping you plan your work more effectively.

By understanding and strategically leveraging hyperfocus, you can turn this unique aspect of ADHD into a powerful asset.

7.2 Diffused Thinking and Creativity

You've probably heard it before, but people with ADHD can have an incredible capacity for creativity. This concept is purely grounded in the way your brain works—individuals with ADHD frequently exhibit high levels of creativity because of their divergent thinking and ability to generate unique ideas.

Divergent thinking is the process of thinking in multiple directions, exploring various possibilities rather than sticking to a single, linear path. This kind of thinking allows you to make unique connections between concepts that might seem unrelated to others. Your brain naturally seeks out novelty and complexity, which can lead to innovative solutions and creative breakthroughs.

Ways to Nurture Creativity

To cultivate this creativity, start by keeping a creativity journal to dedicate space for your ideas, sketches, and inspirations. Carry it with you so that when an idea strikes, you can capture it immediately. Another strategy is to engage in regular brainstorming sessions. Set aside time each week to brainstorm new ideas, whether for work, personal projects, or hobbies. Don't filter your thoughts during these sessions; let your mind roam freely.

Exploring different artistic mediums can also nurture your creativity. Try painting, writing, music, or even digital art—each medium offers a new way to express yourself and can inspire fresh ideas.

Solving Problems with Creativity

Applying your creativity to problem-solving can be a game-changer—and one effective method to apply creativity to problems is by using mind maps to visualize solutions.

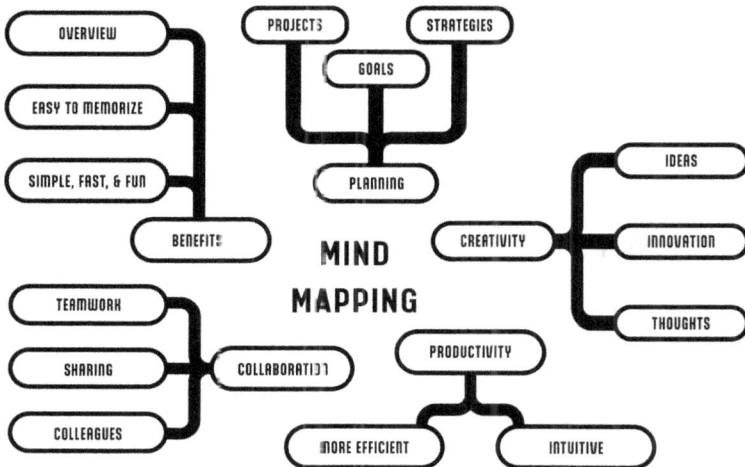

To effectively do mind mapping, start by determining the main problem and placing it in the center of the map, then branch out with different possible solutions, sub-solutions, and related ideas. This visual approach helps you see connections and possibilities that might not be obvious in a linear list.

Not settling for the first solution that comes to mind and approaching problems from multiple angles can also enhance your creative thinking. Considering an issue from different perspectives and thinking about how others might solve it can lead to more comprehensive and innovative solutions.

Sharing Your Creative Work

Showcasing your creative work is just as important as creating it. Building a portfolio of your projects with a physical binder, a digital folder, or a personal website can feel fulfilling, especially when you include your best work, along with notes on your process and inspiration.

Sharing your work in online communities can also be incredibly rewarding. With platforms like Instagram, Behance, and Youtube, if you want to show a more detailed process of your work, that allows you to connect with other creatives, gain feedback, and find inspiration.

Participating in local art exhibitions or events is another excellent way to showcase your work; you can do this by actively looking for community centers, galleries, or even coffee shops that display local artists' work. These venues offer a chance to share your creativity with a broader audience and gain recognition for your talents.

By understanding why individuals with ADHD often exhibit high levels of creativity, you can better appreciate and leverage your own creative potential.

7.3 Problem-Solving Skills

When faced with a problem, your brain doesn't follow the conventional path; instead, it takes a winding road, exploring various possibilities before settling on a solution. This non-linear thinking pattern is a hallmark of ADHD and can be a significant advantage in problem-solving.

While others might see a straight line from point A to point B, you might see multiple routes, each with its own set of opportunities and challenges. This ability to think in different directions allows you to approach problems creatively, finding solutions that others might overlook. Your comfort with ambiguity and complexity further enhances your problem-solving skills. While some might feel overwhelmed by complex issues, you thrive in such environments, seeing them as puzzles to be solved rather than obstacles to be feared.

SCAMPER Technique

To enhance your problem-solving abilities, you can use techniques specifically designed to foster creative thinking. One such technique is SCAMPER, which stands for:

- Substitute
- Combine
- Adapt
- Modify
- Put to another use
- Eliminate
- Reverse

This method encourages you to think about how you can change various aspects of a problem or situation to find a solution, especially in instances when you're working on a project and something isn't working. You may ask yourself what you can substitute or combine to improve it. Could you adapt a method from another field? Can you modify an existing solution to better fit your needs? By systematically exploring these questions, you can generate a range of innovative ideas.

TRIZ Strategy

Another effective technique is TRIZ, or the Theory of Inventive Problem Solving. This method involves identifying and solving contradictions within a problem. For example, you might need a solution that is both strong and lightweight, which seems contradictory at first, but with the framework provided by TRIZ, which is great for resolving such contradictions, you can start drawing on patterns of innovation from various fields can help you break down complex problems into manageable parts and find solutions that balance competing requirements.

Both SCAMPER and TRIZ encourage you to think beyond conventional solutions, leveraging your natural creativity and non-linear thinking.

Collaborating to Solve Problems

Collaborative problem-solving can further enhance your creative abilities. When you work with others, you gain access to diverse perspectives that can lead to innovative solutions, especially when each person brings their unique experiences and ideas to the table, allowing you to build on each other's thoughts.

This collaborative approach can lead to breakthroughs that might not occur in isolation. For instance, in a team setting, one person might identify a potential solution while another refines it, and a third adds a new dimension that makes it even more effective. The synergy created through collaboration can result in solutions that are greater than the sum of their parts.

On a personal note, I recall a time when I faced a challenging situation at work. I was tasked with streamlining a complex process that involved multiple departments. Initially, I felt overwhelmed by the magnitude of the task.

However, by applying creative problem-solving techniques and collaborating with colleagues from different departments, we developed a solution that not only streamlined the process but also improved overall efficiency. We used mind maps to visualize the problem, identify bottlenecks, and brainstorm potential solutions. Each team member contributed their unique insights, and together, we created a more effective workflow. This experience reinforced my belief in the power of creative and collaborative problem-solving.

Embrace your non-linear thinking and comfort with complexity as strengths in problem-solving. Techniques like SCAMPER and TRIZ can help you enhance your creative abilities, while collaborative efforts can lead to innovative solutions. By leveraging these approaches, you can turn challenges into opportunities and find solutions that others might overlook.

7.4 Emotional Intelligence

Living with ADHD often means experiencing emotions more intensely than others. Though this heightened sensitivity can be a double-edged sword, but it also means you might have a deep empathy and an intuitive grasp of others' feelings. Emotional intelligence, or EI, refers to the ability to recognize, understand, and manage our own emotions and those of others.

For adults with ADHD, this can be both a natural strength and an area for growth. Sometimes, you might find that you easily pick up on the emotions of those around you, sensing when someone is upset or stressed even before they say anything. This deep empathy allows you to connect with others on a profound level, fostering strong, meaningful relationships. With proper growth and guidance, your intuitive insights can also guide you in understanding the unspoken needs and desires of others, making you a trusted confidant and a supportive friend.

Honing Emotional Intelligence

Developing emotional intelligence involves several strategies that can enhance your natural abilities. First, practicing active listening is a powerful tool for improving EI. When you listen actively, you focus entirely on the speaker, making eye contact and providing feedback that shows you understand their message. This not only helps you understand others better but also makes them feel valued and heard.

Engaging in self-reflection exercises can also boost your emotional intelligence. Do this by taking time each day to reflect on your emotions and reactions. Ask yourself why you felt a certain way and how you handled the situation to better recognize patterns in your emotional responses, allowing you to manage them more effectively.

Building an emotional vocabulary is another essential step. The better you can articulate your feelings, the easier it is to understand and express them.

Instead of saying you feel "bad," try to describe these emotions more specifically by pinpointing whether you're feeling anxious, frustrated, or disappointed. This precision in language can clarify your emotions and improve your communication.

Using empathy in relationships can significantly enhance your connections with others. One way to do this is by validating others' feelings, which means when someone shares their emotions with you, acknowledge those feelings without judgment. Passing phrases like "I understand why you feel that way" or "It makes sense that you're upset" can go a long way in making others feel understood and supported.

Offering support and understanding by sometimes just being there to listen and provide a shoulder to lean on is enough. Your natural empathetic nature allows you to offer genuine comfort and reassurance, strengthening your bonds with friends and loved ones.

Fine-Tuning Intuition

Intuition plays a vital role in decision-making, especially for those with ADHD. Trusting your gut can guide you through uncertain situations.

When faced with a difficult decision, take a moment to tune into your instincts and ask yourself what feels right or wrong about the options in front of you. This intuitive sense often provides valuable insights that logical analysis might overlook. However, you will still need to balance intuition with rational analysis; while your gut feelings can offer initial guidance, backing them up with facts and logical reasoning ensures well-rounded decisions.

Let's say you have a strong intuition about a business opportunity. Instead of jumping right into making a big decision, take the time to research and gather data to support your instinct. This combination of intuition and rational analysis creates a robust decision-making process.

7.5 Leadership Skills

You may find that your high energy levels and enthusiasm set you apart as a leader. These traits can be absolutely contagious, motivating your team to push through challenges with vigor. When your excitement for a project shows, it becomes a driving force, encouraging others to match your pace and dedication. Your boundless energy can help you tackle multiple tasks, keep morale high, and maintain a dynamic work environment.

Creativity and innovation are other hallmarks of ADHD that can shine in leadership roles. Since you're often able to think outside the box, coming up with novel and effective solutions to problems is almost never a problem. This innovative mindset can be a huge asset in industries that thrive on fresh ideas and forward-thinking approaches. Your ability to see connections that others might miss allows you to create strategies that are both unique and effective. This kind of visionary thinking can propel your team and organization to new heights, setting you apart as a leader who fosters growth and innovation.

The ability to inspire and motivate others is crucial for any leader, and your ADHD traits can enhance this skill. Your passion and enthusiasm can spark a chemical reaction, helping to create a positive and energetic atmosphere, especially when your team sees how invested you are in achieving a goal; they are more likely to commit with the same level of intensity.

Your personal experiences with overcoming challenges can also serve as powerful motivational stories, encouraging your team to persevere and stay focused on their objectives.

Establishing Leadership Skills

Developing leadership skills involves seeking out opportunities for growth. Look for workshops, seminars, or courses that focus on leadership development. These programs often provide practical skills and strategies that you can immediately apply in your role.

Mentorship is another vital component. Find mentors who have experience and knowledge in areas where you wish to grow. Their insights can help you navigate complex situations and make informed decisions, providing a solid foundation for your leadership journey.

Practicing public speaking and presentation skills is another essential aspect of developing as a leader, where effective communication is key to inspiring and guiding your team. Join groups like Toastmasters or take communication courses to build your confidence and hone your public speaking abilities. Regularly practicing in a supportive environment can help you become a more persuasive and engaging speaker, making it easier to convey your vision and rally your team around common goals.

Taking on leadership roles in volunteer organizations can provide valuable hands-on experience. These roles often come with fewer pressures and more flexibility, allowing you to experiment with different leadership styles and strategies, all while providing you a chance to give back to the community and build a sense of fulfillment and purpose. The skills you gain in these roles can easily transfer to your professional life, enhancing your ability to lead and inspire others.

Leading with empathy and understanding is critical for building strong team relationships. Observing empathy allows you to connect with your team members on a personal level, understanding their needs, concerns, and motivations. Creating a strong foundation for this connection fosters trust and loyalty, which encourages a supportive work environment where everyone feels valued.

An inclusive and supportive work environment encourages open communication and collaboration. When team members feel safe and respected, they are more likely to share their ideas and contribute to the team's success.

7.6 Acknowledging Your Strengths

Recognizing the strengths that come with overcoming and leveraging ADHD can be a powerful way to build self-esteem.

Reflecting on your past successes, thinking about the moments when you felt proud of what you achieved, and perhaps even creative projects that received praise, a work task you completed ahead of schedule, or even a personal goal you reached despite the odds.

These accomplishments are not accidents; they are a testament to your unique talents and abilities despite the struggles you face.

Put Your Strengths into Words

It's important to give yourself time to identify these strengths—maybe you're particularly good at thinking on your feet, coming up with creative solutions, or connecting with others on a deep emotional level. Make a conscious effort to not be too hard on yourself and replace negative thoughts with affirmations. For thoughts like "I can never finish anything," counter it with, "I am capable of completing tasks, and I have done it before." Practice self-gratitude by acknowledging your personal strengths.

So, for each evening, jot down a few things you did well that day. They don't have to be monumental achievements; even small victories count, like making your bed or washing the dishes instead of leaving them on the sink for another day. Writing these strengths down and revisiting the list whenever self-doubt creeps in is a tangible reminder of what you're capable of. This practice helps shift your focus from what you didn't do to what you did accomplish, fostering a more positive self-view.

Acknowledge and Remind Yourself

Building that confidence through your strengths involves setting and achieving small goals. Of course, this means that you should start with something manageable, like organizing a small part of your workspace or completing a task you've been putting off—*don't* directly jump into a larger task; start slow. Providing yourself with a sense of accomplishment by achieving these small goals can build momentum. Each milestone you reach, no matter how small, is a step towards greater confidence.

Never forget to acknowledge your wins, whether it's by treating yourself to something you enjoy or simply taking a moment to reflect on your success. These moments reinforce positive behavior. If acknowledging and celebrating *each* achievement sounds a bit much, then you can always stick to celebrating the accomplishment of tasks you found great difficulty in—or when you finish a set number of "completed tasks."

Share Your Goals for Celebration, Not Just for Validation

In times of self-doubt, an outside perspective can highlight strengths you might overlook, so when you share your goals and achievements with friends, family, or colleagues who support you, their encouragement can be a powerful motivator. You can celebrate your wins and strengths with them this way.

It's normal to seek validation, and sometimes, having this type of validation can be healthy, but when you *constantly seek* validation, it can backfire and potentially hurt you when done excessively. This does **not** mean that you should push your peers away to force yourself to validate and celebrate by yourself; instead, take a *pause* and read what you've written for yourself. As mentioned in Chapter 5, showing self-love and compassion is extremely important. Share your goals when you want to celebrate, and not just for the validation.

ADHD is not a flaw but a different way of thinking. Shifting your mindset by acknowledging that your brain processes information in unique ways, which can be a strength in many situations, is a sign of self-acceptance and self-love.

Advocate for yourself by communicating your needs and strengths to others; when you need a quiet workspace to focus or regular breaks to stay productive, don't hesitate to ask for these accommodations.

Additionally, advocate for others with ADHD. Share your experiences and insights to help dispel myths and promote understanding. This not only benefits the ADHD community but also reinforces your own acceptance and pride in your identity. Take a moment to acknowledge your journey and the strengths you've developed along the way.

By recognizing your unique talents, practicing positive self-talk, building confidence through small goals, and embracing neurodiversity, you can foster a strong sense of self-esteem.

Overcome each and every challenge, and allow yourself to shine brightest with everything that you can achieve.

Reflective Exercise: Identifying and Overcoming Obstacles

Try to answer these reflection questions:

- What potential barriers might hinder my progress?
- How can I develop contingency plans to address these barriers?
- Who can I seek support from to stay accountable and motivated?

Take a moment to reflect on these questions and jot down your thoughts. Identifying obstacles and planning for them can significantly increase your chances of achieving your long-term goals. Consider discussing your reflections with a mentor or accountability partner for additional insights and support.

By setting and achieving long-term goals, you create a roadmap for your future. This roadmap provides direction, enhances motivation, and helps you navigate the complexities of life with ADHD. Remember, the key to success lies in breaking down larger goals into manageable steps, tracking your progress, and seeking support when needed.

As you work towards your goals, you'll discover a newfound sense of purpose and accomplishment, empowering you to thrive despite the challenges of ADHD.

Chapter 8

Nurturing Positive Lifestyle Changes

After a long day, it's tempting to grab whatever snack is closest or sink into the couch without moving for hours. But have you ever paused to consider how these daily choices impact your ADHD symptoms?

Skipping movement, missing a workout, or relying on sugary snacks and processed foods can leave you feeling even more scattered and fatigued, amplifying the challenges you already face.

Both nutrition and lifestyle habits play a significant role in managing ADHD. What you eat and how you structure your day can influence your mood, energy levels, and ability to focus.

By understanding the powerful connection between your diet, physical activity, and mental clarity, you can take meaningful steps to improve your daily life and better manage your symptoms.

8.1 Nutrition and ADHD

The way nutrition impacts ADHD is quite simple: it starts with blood sugar levels. When you consume foods high in sugar, your blood sugar spikes, giving you a quick burst of energy. However, this spike is often followed by a crash, leaving you feeling tired, irritable, and unable to concentrate, which can heavily affect the way you work, study, or even do your hobbies.

Essential Nutrients

Stabilizing your blood sugar levels is an absolute priority in managing mood and focus, so consuming foods rich in complex carbohydrates, like whole grains, can help keep your blood sugar steady, providing a consistent source of energy throughout the day.

Incorporating the right foods into your diet, such as those rich in Omega-3 (e.g., salmon and flaxseeds), is known to support brain health and improve cognitive function. These fatty acids maintain the structure and function of brain cells, aiding in better focus and attention. Whole grains, like brown rice and oatmeal, provide steady energy, preventing blood sugar spikes that can lead to mood swings and decreased concentration.

Meanwhile, high-protein snacks, such as nuts and seeds, offer sustained energy and help stabilize blood sugar levels. Protein is essential for the production of neurotransmitters, which are chemicals that transmit signals in the brain, aiding in better focus and mood regulation.

On the flip side, certain foods can intensify ADHD symptoms. Sugary snacks and drinks are highly addictive and are some of the biggest culprits. They could provide a quick energy boost, but it's often followed by a sharp decline, leaving you feeling sluggish and unfocused. Caffeine, found in coffee, tea, and many sodas, can also be addictive and impact hyperactivity. While some adults with ADHD find that small amounts of caffeine help them focus, excessive consumption can lead to increased restlessness and anxiety.

Many processed foods also contain artificial colors and flavors—artificial additives and preservatives—which can exacerbate symptoms. Studies have shown that these additives can increase hyperactivity and impulsivity in some individuals.

Reducing these negative effects and improving your overall well-being means that you need to *actively* avoid processed foods; and choose natural, whole foods instead. Minimizing unhealthy processed foods in your diet will help you improve the way you manage your ADHD symptoms more effectively.

Planning your meals with these considerations in mind can set you up for success. Preparing healthy snacks in advance can prevent you from reaching for convenient but unhealthy options. Keep a stash of nuts, seeds, and fresh fruits within easy reach. Creating a weekly meal plan can help you stay organized and ensure you're consuming a balanced diet. Include a variety of fruits and vegetables to provide essential vitamins and minerals that support brain function.

Batch-cooking meals and storing them in individual portions can save time and reduce the temptation to opt for fast food or processed snacks.

Personalizing Your Nutrition Plan

Note down the meals and eating patterns you observe, and consider how you can incorporate more brain-healthy foods into your diet. Create a simple meal plan for the week ahead, focusing on incorporating whole grains, high-protein snacks, and omega-3-rich foods. You may also want to speak with a dietician to understand more about your diet. Once you've set your plans and executed them, observe how these changes impact your mood and ability to focus.

Making informed choices that support your overall well-being once you understand the connection between ADHD and nutrition and making small changes in your diet can lead to significant improvements in managing your ADHD symptoms, helping you feel more balanced, focused, and energized.

8.2 Physical and Recreational Activities

Restless nights with your mind buzzing and focus out of reach can feel all too familiar. But what if you started your day differently? Imagine stepping outside for a refreshing morning walk, gliding through the pool for a few calming laps, or capturing the beauty of the world through a lens while exploring your surroundings. Channeling restless energy into purposeful movement not only grounds your thoughts but also transforms how you feel and function throughout the day.

Managing ADHD symptoms isn't just about focusing on what's going on internally; there are also external factors that promote focus, attention, and, most of all, increase dopamine levels. Physically moving yourself by engaging in any form of exercise regularly can improve your overall concentration, allowing you to tackle tasks with greater clarity.

Exercise stimulates the release of neurotransmitters like dopamine and norepinephrine, which allow you to improve attention and mood regulation. This direct boost in brain chemicals helps reduce impulsivity and hyperactivity, making it easier to stay on task. Additionally, exercise enhances mood and reduces anxiety—the endorphins released during physical activity act as natural mood lifters, helping to combat feelings of stress and overwhelm.

Aerobic Exercises

Certain types of exercise are particularly beneficial for ADHD. Aerobic exercises, such as running, swimming, and cycling, are excellent choices. These activities increase your heart rate and promote better blood flow to the brain, enhancing cognitive function.

Running through a park or swimming in a pool can provide a sense of rhythm and calm, helping to soothe a restless mind.

Strength Training

Strength training is another valuable addition to your exercise routine. Lifting weights or doing bodyweight exercises like push-ups and squats can improve overall health and build physical strength. Strength training also requires focus and discipline, which can help develop better self-control and reduce impulsivity.

Yoga and Mindfulness

Yoga and mindfulness practices offer a unique combination of physical movement and mental relaxation. The slow, deliberate movements and deep breathing exercises in yoga can improve flexibility and reduce stress. Mindfulness practices, often integrated into yoga, teach you to stay present and manage your thoughts, providing a powerful tool for emotional regulation.

Creating and maintaining an exercise routine would sound exhausting, but breaking it down into smaller steps can make it more achievable. Setting clear and realistic fitness goals, whether it's running a certain distance, lifting a specific weight, or practicing yoga for a set amount of time, can provide motivation and direction. You can even mix it up a bit with a variety of activities to prevent boredom. Doing aerobic exercises with strength training and following it up with yoga ensures that your routine stays interesting and engaging.

If running feels monotonous one day, switch it up with a swim or a yoga session. You can even try to find a workout buddy or join a class or a gym boot camp (if you're ready for it), which can also make a significant difference.

Having a trustworthy companion or friend to exercise with provides accountability and makes the activity more enjoyable. Even group classes, whether in person or online, offer a sense of community and support, making it easier to stay committed.

And, if you're worried about being judged at the gym, don't be. Gymgoers are just like you—they're focused on their own exercises and workout routines and will tend to mind their own business, but they're also quite helpful, with some even providing tips if you're unsure of what you should do next.

For most adults, however, time management and overcoming barriers to exercise are common challenges. When you're fitting workouts into your busy schedule, try breaking them into shorter sessions throughout the day.

Most would say that you would need to exercise a full 2 hours at least—but for those with a hectic schedule, a simple 10-minute run in the morning, a quick strength training session around noon, and yoga practice in the evening can add up to a comprehensive routine and allow you to build a less sedentary lifestyle.

Considering that these exercises *can* get a little monotonous and boring, making exercise enjoyable is another key to consistency. Choose activities that you genuinely enjoy and look forward to. If you love dancing, incorporate it into your routine.

If you find peace in nature, opt for outdoor activities like hiking or cycling. Dealing with motivation issues can be tricky, but allowing yourself to do and complete small, achievable goals and celebrating your progress can really help.

Tracking your workouts in a journal or using a fitness app can provide a sense of accomplishment and keep you motivated. A smart fitness watch can also help you keep a more detailed track of your progress.

Other Recreational Activities

Aside from exercise and other physical activities, one can get into different hobbies to keep your mind active and energy well-spent—with the added benefit of honing your more creative side.

Hobbies are more than just leisure activities—they offer a sense of achievement and a creative outlet that helps reduce stress and manage ADHD symptoms. Whether it's painting, writing, or learning a new dance move, hobbies provide fulfillment by channeling energy into something enjoyable and productive. The right hobbies can be transformative, allowing hyperfocus and deep engagement that is both relaxing and stimulating.

Physical activities like hiking or dancing not only reduce hyperactivity but also improve focus, while group hobbies like book clubs or sports foster social connections and combat isolation. Choose activities that align with your interests and provide a mix of solitary and social engagement.

Balancing hobbies with responsibilities requires a bit of planning. Schedule hobby time as a priority while ensuring important tasks, like work or chores, are completed first. For instance, you might finish your workday before dedicating an hour to painting. This approach ensures a healthy balance between obligations and leisure.

Exploring new hobbies can keep life exciting. Going through community classes, workshops, and hobby groups lets you discover new interests and meet like-minded people. Whether it's pottery, cooking, or photography, trying new activities can reveal hidden talents and passions. Don't be afraid to step out of your comfort zone—you might find immense joy and fulfillment in something entirely unexpected.

All of these different activities offer a multitude of cognitive and emotional benefits for managing ADHD. Improved focus, reduced impulsivity, enhanced mood, and decreased anxiety are just a few of the positive outcomes.

Incorporating aerobic exercises, strength training, and yoga into your routine provides a well-rounded approach to physical activity, and engaging in different hobbies can help you express yourself in a more fun and sometimes challenging way.

By setting realistic goals, incorporating variety, finding support, and overcoming common barriers, you can create and maintain an exercise and hobby routine that supports your ADHD management and overall well-being.

8.3 Creating a Calming Environment

A common problem among those with ADHD is exposure to cluttered, noisy, or overstimulating spaces. A calm and quiet environment is often needed by those with ADHD, as spaces that are full of potential distractions can make it harder to focus, worsen symptoms, and may even leave you feeling overwhelmed. By creating a calming environment, you can reduce and prevent overstimulation while promoting relaxation and focus.

Imagine walking into a room painted in soothing blues and greens, with minimal clutter and soft lighting. An area like this can invite calm and help your mind settle, making it easier to concentrate on tasks or unwind after a long day.

Decluttering Distractions

Environmental distractions, like noise from a busy street or a cluttered room, can make it hard to concentrate. Digital distractions, such as social media notifications or incoming emails, are just as disruptive. Internal distractions, like intrusive thoughts or daydreaming, can sap your focus without realizing it.

So, decluttering and organizing common areas will lessen the impact of visual distractions while allowing you to find the things you need easily. If you have too many small objects scattered around, consider using storage solutions like bins and shelves to keep items organized and out of sight. Doing this isn't a one-time activity; it's a continuous process that takes time to build into a solid habit for those with ADHD.

If you're unsure of how or where to start decluttering, you can try the *KonMari Method*, which was developed and popularized by Marie Kondo in 2014. The whole idea of this method is to sort your items into categories rather than by location. Hold each item and ask yourself if it *sparks joy*—if it doesn't, thank it for its service and let it go.

Building a regular decluttering routine can help maintain an organized space. Set aside time each week to go through your belongings and get rid of what you no longer need. This habit prevents clutter from accumulating and keeps your environment functional and pleasant.

With the right approach, you can turn chaos into order and make your spaces work for you, not against you—regularly decluttering your home can prevent messes from accumulating and maintain a serene environment.

Sensory-Friendly Additions

Another element to consider when building a calming environment is the sensory considerations. **Soft lighting** options, such as dimmable lamps or LED lights, can reduce glare and create a more comfortable atmosphere. Harsh, bright lights can be overstimulating, while softer lighting can help you feel more relaxed and focused.

Aromatherapy with calming scents like lavender can also contribute to a soothing environment. Using essential oil diffusers is a simple way to introduce these scents into your space. Lavender, chamomile, and sandalwood are known for their relaxing properties and can help reduce stress and anxiety.

White noise machines or apps can provide a consistent background sound that drowns out other noises. The gentle hum of white noise can create a more stable auditory environment, helping you concentrate better and sleep more soundly. If you prefer to have no noise, you can try going for noise-canceling headphones or comfortable ear muffs to muffle sounds.

Home Optimization

Think about the different areas of your home and how you can make each one more ADHD-friendly, like the bedroom. Not only will you be establishing a bedtime and wake-up routine to help regulate your sleep patterns, you can also try to make your bedroom more sleep-friendly.

Use soft, neutral colors and eliminate clutter to create a restful space. Using calming colors like pale blues and greens has also been shown to reduce stress and create a sense of tranquility. And when you add natural elements like plants into the room, it can also enhance the calming effect while improving air quality and bringing a touch of nature indoors, which can be soothing. Taking it a step further, you could also make the bedroom a no-electronics zone to reduce distractions and promote better sleep.

As for the bathroom, keep daily items in baskets or bins for easy access, and consider using soothing essential oils during your bath or shower to create a relaxing experience. Setting a timer can prevent you from procrastinating in the bathroom and help you stay on schedule. Maybe try to keep this area a no-electronics zone as well.

In the kitchen, maintain organization with a weekly menu and grocery list. Designate specific areas for food prep, serving, and dirty dishes to streamline your cooking process. Make it a habit to keep countertops clear of unnecessary items once you're done preparing your meals. Spend a few minutes each week organizing your cupboards to ensure everything is easy to find.

If you have an exercise room, create a dedicated space with soothing colors and essential equipment like weights, a treadmill, and a yoga mat. A large mirror can help you focus on your movements and make the space feel larger.

Workspace Considerations

Other than your home, optimizing your workspace is just as important. Going for ergonomic furniture like a good chair for your back and a desk at the right height can make a great difference in your comfort and productivity by promoting proper posture and lessening physical strain to allow you to work more efficiently.

A minimalist desk setup would mean that you only get to keep the essential items on your desk and store everything else in drawers or shelves; keeping a whiteboard bulletin board or wall calendar for scheduling would be ideal. This can prevent visual clutter and help you concentrate on the task at hand.

Using noise-canceling headphones can block out background noise, creating a quieter workspace. Auditory distractions, whether you work from home or in an office, can also improve your ability to focus. And if you live with family members, communicating with family members in advance about minimizing interruptions when you're working—even hanging up a sign outside your door—can help prevent distractions.

A stress-free environment is crucial for self-care in managing ADHD. Knowing when to take breaks and redirect your attention can help maintain a calm household.

8.4 Financial Management

Managing finances can be an exhausting and anxiety-riddled task for *any* adult, especially when ADHD can add layers of complexity to tracking expenses, saving, and budgeting.

Impulsive spending is one of the most common financial challenges. You might find yourself making spontaneous purchases, only to regret them later. These impulses can quickly add up, leaving a dent in your budget and creating unnecessary stress later in the month, usually until the next payday.

Difficulty tracking expenses is another hurdle. Keeping tabs on where your money goes each month can feel like trying to catch water with a sieve. You might forget to record transactions or lose track of receipts, leading to an incomplete picture of your finances.

Challenges with saving and budgeting compound these issues. Setting aside money for future needs requires practicing frugality, discipline, and forward planning, all of which can be particularly challenging when ADHD is in the mix.

Creating a realistic and effective budget starts with listing all your income sources and expenses. This includes your salary, freelance income, and any other sources of money you receive.

Once you have a clear picture of your income, categorize your expenses into fixed, variable, and discretionary categories.

Here are some notes to help you determine which categories to put your expenses in:

- **Fixed expenses** are those that remain constant each month, like rent or mortgage payments, utilities, and insurance.
- **Variable expenses** fluctuate, such as groceries, gas, and entertainment.
- **Discretionary expenses** are non-essential, like dining out or buying new clothes.

By categorizing your expenses, you can see where your money is going and identify areas where you can cut back. Setting savings goals is an essential part of budgeting. Whether it's building an emergency fund, saving for a vacation, or planning for retirement, having clear goals can provide motivation and direction.

Determine how much you want to save each month and treat it as a fixed expense. This way, you prioritize saving and make it a regular part of your financial routine.

To assist with budgeting and financial management, several tools and apps can make the process more manageable.

Financial Strategies

Managing impulsive spending requires specific strategies to keep your finances in check. One effective technique is implementing a 24-hour rule before making purchases.

When you feel the urge to buy something, wait for 24 hours before making the decision. This pause allows you to reflect on whether the purchase is necessary and helps curb impulsive behavior.

Using cash instead of credit cards can also limit impulsive buying. When you pay with cash, you physically see the money leaving your hands, which can make you more mindful (and hopefully more discouraged) of your spending.

Set spending limits for different categories to prevent overspending. For example, allocate a specific amount for dining out each month and stick to it. This approach helps you stay within your budget and avoid financial stress.

Checking Your Financial Habits

Create a simple action plan to address your financial challenges. For example, if you find yourself overspending on dining out, plan to cook more meals at home and allocate a portion of your budget to groceries.

Track your progress and celebrate small victories along the way. Each step you take towards better financial management brings you closer to achieving your goals and reducing financial stress.

8.5 Travel Tips

Traveling can be both exciting and nerve-wracking, especially when ADHD is part of the equation. Thankfully, minimizing travel stress and managing your symptoms lies in preparation.

Creating a detailed itinerary for a long trip is an incredibly effective way to outline your travel plans, which include flight times, hotel check-ins, activities, and probably even restaurants.

Once you have your itinerary, you can break it down into manageable chunks, allowing you to anticipate what's next without feeling overwhelmed. And on the topic of hotel check-ins, researching accommodations and amenities in advance can save you a lot of headaches. Look for hotels that offer quiet rooms, free breakfast, or easy access to public transport. Knowing what to expect can make your stay more comfortable and less stressful.

Another important list is the packing checklists. List everything you need, from clothes to toiletries to medications. This helps ensure you don't forget essentials, reduce last-minute panic, and avoid the potential rush of repeatedly checking your hand-carry for said essentials.

On the day you do start traveling, managing time and schedules during your trip requires some strategic planning. Setting alarms and reminders for important activities ensures you stay on track. Use your phone or a travel app to set reminders for flight departures, excursions, and even mealtimes; doing so can help you avoid the last-minute anxiety rush and keep your day running smoothly.

Travel apps for real-time updates are invaluable. Navigation or map apps can provide real-time information on flight delays, traffic conditions, and public transportation schedules. This keeps you informed and allows you to adjust plans if needed. Allowing extra time for transitions and delays is another smart move. However, travel often comes with unexpected hiccups, so build buffer time between activities. If your flight lands at 3 PM, don't schedule a dinner reservation for 4 PM. Give yourself a cushion to handle any unforeseen delays—it *can* happen.

Staying organized on the go can make a world of difference. Using packing cubes for organization helps you keep your suitcase tidy and makes it easier to find items. Assign different cubes for different categories, such as clothes, toiletries, and gadgets. Keeping important documents in a dedicated pouch ensures you can quickly access your passport, boarding passes, and hotel reservations, which minimizes the risk of losing vital documents and reduces anxiety.

Maintaining a travel journal or digital log can also be beneficial. Note down or print out your itinerary, important contact numbers, and any other critical information. This serves as a handy reference and helps you stay organized throughout your trip.

Enjoying and relaxing during travel is as important as staying organized. Practicing mindfulness each day—taking deep breaths and focusing on your surroundings—can ground you and reduce stress. Immerse yourself in local activities, like visiting markets, trying regional dishes, or attending cultural events, to enrich your journey.

Balance sightseeing with downtime to recharge and prevent burnout. Schedule moments to unwind, whether lounging, reading, or taking a leisurely walk.

Traveling with ADHD becomes manageable and fulfilling with preparation, organization, and a focus on enjoyment. These steps reduce stress, allowing you to fully embrace the adventure and create lasting memories.

Conclusion

As we conclude this journey, let's reflect on the core message of this book: living with ADHD is not a limitation but an opportunity to grow, adapt, and thrive.

This guide was created to offer practical tools, strategies, and insights to help you navigate challenges and harness your unique strengths.

From understanding the complexities of ADHD to implementing time management, relationship-building, and self-care strategies, the goal is to empower you with knowledge and actionable steps. Each chapter highlights ways to enhance your daily life, manage relationships, and build a supportive lifestyle that fosters well-being and resilience.

Remember, managing ADHD is a continuous process. Progress may be slow at times, but every step forward counts. Be patient with yourself, embrace self-compassion, and celebrate your achievements—no matter how small. Stay informed, connect with others in the ADHD community, and keep exploring strategies that work for you.

This journey is not about perfection but about growth, self-discovery, and creating a fulfilling life on your terms.

Thank you for taking the time to invest in yourself through this book. Your commitment to understanding and managing

ADHD is a testament to your strength and potential. Embrace your unique journey, and know that you have the tools to succeed and thrive.

Here's to a life of empowerment, growth, and fulfillment— your best life awaits.

-     *Kate Winslow*

Empowering Others on the ADHD Journey

Now that you have the tools and strategies to embrace your ADHD and thrive, it's time to share your experience and help others find the same support and insights.

By leaving your honest review of this book on Amazon, you'll guide other adults with ADHD, their families, and supporters to the resources they need to better understand and manage the condition. Your review can be the first step for someone else to take control of their life and feel empowered in their journey.

Thank you for your time and support. The conversation around ADHD grows stronger when we share knowledge and experiences – and you're helping to make a difference.

With gratitude,
Kate Winslow

References

10 Best ADHD Productivity Software Tools & Apps 2024
https://clickup.com/blog/adhd-productivity-tools/

32 of the Best Ways to Get Organized When You Have ADHD
https://psychcentral.com/adhd/the-best-ways-to-get-
organized-when-you-have-adhd

9 Tips for Creating a Routine for Adults with ADHD
https://psychcentral.com/adhd/9-tips-for-creating-a-
routine-for-adults-with-adhd

ADHD and Exercise: What You Need to Know
https://www.healthline.com/health/fitness/adhd-and-
exercise

ADHD and Focus: Effective Strategies to Reduce Distractions
https://www.theminiadhdcoach.com/adhd-symptoms/adhd-
distractions

ADHD Can Strain Relationships. Here's How Couples Cope.
https://www.nytimes.com/2022/02/18/well/mind/adhd-
dating-relationships.html

ADHD Emotional Dysregulation: Managing Intense Emotions
https://add.org/emotional-dysregulation-adhd/

ADHD Memory Loss: Science-Backed Ways to Boost Your ...
https://add.org/adhd-memory-loss/

ADHD Research Roundup: December 15, 2023
https://www.psychiatrictimes.com/view/adhd-research-
roundup-december-15-2023

Anxiety disorders in adult ADHD: A frequent comorbidity ...
https://www.sciencedirect.com/science/article/pii/S01651781
22000373

Best Mental Health Apps for ADHD
    https://www.additudemag.com/slideshows/best-mental-
    health-apps-for-adhd-headspace-talkspace-better-help/

Building Resilience: How Cognitive Flexibility and ...
    https://effectiveeffortconsulting.com/building-resilience-
    how-cognitive-flexibility-and-emotional-regulation-
    empower-adhd-individuals/

Chunking: Breaking Tasks into Manageable Parts
    https://www.neverdefeatedcoaching.net/chunking-
    breaking-tasks-into-manageable-parts/

Creativity and ADHD: A review of behavioral studies, the ...
    https://pubmed.ncbi.nlm.nih.gov/33035524/

Depression and ADHD: How They're Linked - WebMD
    https://www.webmd.com/add-adhd/depression-adhd-link

Eating Patterns and Dietary Interventions in ADHD
    https://www.ncbi.nlm.nih.gov/pmc/articles/PMC9608000/

Genetics of ADHD: What Should the Clinician Know? - PMC
    https://www.ncbi.nlm.nih.gov/pmc/articles/PMC7046577/

How Can Family Members, Friends, and Partners Better ...
    https://www.envisionadhd.com/single-post/how-can-
    family-members-friends-and-partners-better-understand-
    and-support-an-adult-with-adhd

How Cognitive Behavioral Therapy Can Help Manage ADHD
    https://www.healthline.com/health/adhd/cbt-for-adhd

How to Create a Calm Home for People with ADHD
    https://www.addrc.org/how-to-create-a-calm-home-for-
    people-with-adhd/

How to Create SMART Goals - Next Step 4 ADHD
    https://nextstep4adhd.com/how-to-create-smart-goals/

How to Create SMART Goals https://nextstep4adhd.com/how-to-
    create-smart-goals/

How to Practice Self Compassion with ADHD
https://www.additudemag.com/self-compassion-practice-adhd-shame/

Hyperfocus: the forgotten frontier of attention - PMC
https://www.ncbi.nlm.nih.gov/pmc/articles/PMC7851038/

Managing Money and ADHD: Expenses and Goals
https://chadd.org/for-adults/managing-money-and-adhd-expenses-and-goals/

Social Anxiety and ADHD: How to better manage ...
https://drsharonsaline.com/2021/10/19/social-anxiety-and-adhd-how-to-better-manage-anxiety-with-supportive-planning-and-preparation/

Survive And Thrive With ADHD Leadership
https://www.forbes.com/sites/drnancydoyle/2020/02/23/survive-and-thrive-with-adhd-leadership-everything-you-need-to-know-from-a-ceo-whos-been-there/

The brain anatomy of attention-deficit/hyperactivity disorder ...
https://www.ncbi.nlm.nih.gov/pmc/articles/PMC5391018/

Time Management Skills for ADHD Brains: Practical Advice
https://www.additudemag.com/time-management-skills-adhd-brain/

Understanding ADHD and How Emotional Intelligence May ...
https://www.ei-magazine.com/post/understanding-adhd-and-how-emotional-intelligence-may-help-to-alleviate-the-symptoms

Unveiling Effective ADHD Communication Strategies
https://justmind.org/adhd-communication-strategies/

What Is Executive Function? 7 Deficits Tied to ADHD
https://www.additudemag.com/7-executive-function-deficits-linked-to-adhd/